Praise for

the fab mom's
G U I D E

"I don't know anyone else more passionate about helping women keep it together in the throes of new motherhood—Jill cracks the code for any new mom who wants to bounce back!"
—Ali Landry, actress, television host, and cofounder of Celebrity Red Carpet Safety Event

"In this book, Jill offers creative suggestions for new moms that make us feel like 'us' again. Her humor, refreshing honesty and personal stories will stick with you."
—Debbie Matenopoulos, cohost of Hallmark's *Home & Family*, cohost of *The Insider* on CBS, and bestselling cookbook author

"*The FAB Mom's Guide* solves the challenging issues for first-time mothers—things I wish I would've read about when I was pregnant. It's a must-read for any new mom!"
—Jenn Brown, two-time Emmy Award winning sportscaster & television host

"We had so much fun reading *The FAB Mom's Guide*. Jill's warm charm jumps right off the page."
—Erin & Ian Ziering, AtHomeWithTheZierings.com

"Jill Simonian always manages to be totally honest, hysterically funny, *and* inspirational when she's talking about babies, parenting, and getting your mom groove back."
—Rebecca Dube, NBC's *TODAY Show* parenting team editor

"Jill Simonian is the girlfriend every new mom needs—with helpful tips and her trademark humor, she'll get you through the first few months of parenting in style."

—Megan Sayers, senior editor at Babble.com

"Jill has a special and very approachable way of connecting. . . Her willingness to share real-life experiences really empowers new moms."

—Becky Talley, editorial and social media manager for Right Start Baby

"*The FAB Mom* is an honest and *hilarious* book that feels like it was written by your best friend... If there's anyone who can make wearing a postpartum diaper feel fab, it's Jill!"

—Emma Bing, lifestyle editor at WhatToExpect.com and daughter of *What to Expect . . .* book series author Heidi Murkoff

"Authentic, approachable, and encouraging, Jill provides comfort (with a side of humor!) as we face pressures and the sometimes challenging decisions we must make as new moms. I wish this book was around when I became a mom six years ago! This is a perfect read for any new mom who needs to be reminded that she is doing her very best and that she too will bounce back!"

—Lindsay Pinchuk, founder and CEO of Bump Club and Beyond

"Jill Simonian is one of very favorite mom writers! She's funny and smart—the kind of woman you want to sit down and have a glass of wine with. She dishes on motherhood in all its awesome craziness and we so appreciate her honesty."

—Cerentha Harris, editor of Mom.me

the fab mom's
G U I D E
How to Get Over the Bump
& Bounce Back Fast After Baby

Jill Simonian

Skyhorse Publishing

Copyright © 2017 by Jill Simonian
Illustrations © 2017 by Anne Higgins Clark

All rights reserved. No part of this book may be reproduced in any manner without the express written consent of the publisher, except in the case of brief excerpts in critical reviews or articles. All inquiries should be addressed to Skyhorse Publishing, 307 West 36th Street, 11th Floor, New York, NY 10018.

Skyhorse Publishing books may be purchased in bulk at special discounts for sales promotion, corporate gifts, fund-raising, or educational purposes. Special editions can also be created to specifications. For details, contact the Special Sales Department, Skyhorse Publishing, 307 West 36th Street, 11th Floor, New York, NY 10018 or info@skyhorsepublishing.com.

Skyhorse® and Skyhorse Publishing® are registered trademarks of Skyhorse Publishing, Inc.®, a Delaware corporation.

Visit our website at www.skyhorsepublishing.com.

10 9 8 7 6 5 4 3 2 1

Library of Congress Cataloging-in-Publication Data is available on file.

Cover design by Jane Sheppard
Cover photo credit: Anne Keenan Higgins

Print ISBN: 978-1-5107-1516-5
Ebook ISBN: 978-1-5107-1518-9

Printed in China

To

Leah and Samantha (my girls),
You are the most fabulous little women I know.

Bonnie (my mom),
You're the most FAB of all and always keep my head on straight.

CONTENTS

NOTE TO READERS

This book is designed to help you make informed decisions about your lifestyle. Information given here are the ideas of its author, who is not a trained medical, health, fitness, psychology, or psychiatric professional. The ideas in this book are not intended to diagnose, treat, cure, or prevent any kind of medical or psychiatric problem or condition. If you have a condition that requires care, please seek treatment from your healthcare provider.

The opinions provided in this book are not intended to replace the advice of qualified health professionals in any way, but are rather provided for informational and entertainment purposes only. The author and experts featured in this book disclaim all responsibility for, and are not liable for, any liability, loss, or risk, personal or otherwise, which is incurred as a consequence, directly or indirectly, of the use and application in any of the contents of this book.

Products featured in this book are copyright and trademarks of their respective owners. None of these owners have sponsored, authorized, or endorsed this book in any way. Unless noted, author and experts are not affiliated with brands or products mentioned in this book.

AN INTRODUCTION . . .

Congratulations! You're having a baby. (Or maybe you've just had a baby?) Cheers. Well done. Get it, girl. I'm guessing you want to bounce back fast? Welcome to the club, ambitious woman. Between high-powered working moms, new celebrity moms on Instagram, rock star homemaker moms, and that random chick from your gym who was exercising up until the very day of her own delivery, bouncing back fast after having a baby is something a lot of us fantasize about during the nine months leading up to the big reveal (I did, anyway). Bouncing back fast can also be a realistic and empowering thing if you opt to do it without hesitation.

As someone who now finds herself working as a parenting lifestyle contributor and expert in media, I'm the first to scream about how easy it is to get confused and frustrated with today's overabundant advice about how to have our babies and raise our kids and the best ways to take care of ourselves. Thanks to social media, there's this crazy notion that we all live the most fabulous lives without much fault. (Spare me the facade.) Since we're going

1

to spend serious time together and spill secrets for how to truly become a "fab mom," I need to come clean: being a FAB Mom doesn't mean looking like a zillion bucks all the time (like the "fab" nickname leads you to believe).

The key to being a FAB mom and feeling more secure and happy the first year with baby depends on readjusting and recentering your *focus*. Bouncing back and conquering new motherhood on a day-to-day basis depends on a new mom's ability to think clearly from the inside, rather than just looking fabulous on the outside. About 80 percent of new moms experience natural baby blues and mood swings after having a baby—many of these feelings are linked to a change in identity. *(I'm a mom now?! What the heck am I supposed to do? Who am I?)* So yes, the big *aha*-moment here is that FAB is actually an acronym: Focused After Baby. (Get it? F-A-B! Ha.) Don't feel tricked—and please don't take this book back! We're going to have a blast.

The focus, moxie, and directions to a more fulfilled sense of self you will discover and hopefully follow in this guide will lead to surprising revelations, inspired perspective, and practical know-how that's going to rock your new life as a mom. Hell, it's going to rock your life as a *woman*. I'm betting right now that you're soon going to be very impressed with yourself after having a baby . . . regardless of how organized and together you may already be.

This book isn't going to outline every phase of your pregnancy, tell you how big your baby is at the midway mark, or describe all the scientific details about what happens to your body during and after birth. You can find all that stuff online or in other books and talk about it with your girlfriends. This book is about making choices that will spawn resilience and an invigorating approach to new mom life so that you can be a better you beginning with the birth of your baby. You just might find yourself reinvented and better after baby.

The personal tips I share are not without faults and trade-offs, but they're honest, authentic, practical, inexpensive, and all tried and tested by yours truly—it's up to you to decide which costs are cool with you to cope with and which costs you can't bear to pay. The combination of lifestyle choices in this book worked effectively for me through two back-to-back pregnancies and births within two years while I launched a new brand (my blog, TheFABMom. com) and continued to build a competitive career in media. Most tips—or, maybe all—will most likely work for you, too. Do a few of them seem shallow? Yes. Are some of them unpopular with the contemporary parenting crowd? Yes. But, if followed as described in this book, these tricks will bounce you back quickly after having a baby and give you the foundation and tools to be a FAB mom in mind, body, and spirit as your baby grows.

Why bother writing this guide in the first place? Well, when I was expecting my first baby, I couldn't find another resource like it. (Trust me, I looked!) Since I couldn't find any books, articles, or real people that could offer me insight and inspiration back then, I started spontaneously inventing my own program of choices and to-dos to see what stuck, what didn't, and if this crazy notion of bouncing back fast was even possible in the first place. What did I find? I found it was possible. I also found myself feeling more powerful, more fun, more productive, more fulfilled, more joyous, and more manageable—not only for the first year of baby's life, but for the preschool and early school years that have followed.

You don't need a night nurse. You don't need a nanny. You don't need a personal trainer. But, there are controversial choices involving your boobs and breast milk to contend with. There are shameless rituals involving your underwear. There are activities to be done naked against your bathroom sink before you brush your teeth. It's not a cakewalk. There are choices and costs, but each story, suggestion, and trick has a larger purpose attached to it: to make you more resilient for the frequent, head-spinning, everyday life challenges that new motherhood brings.

You might react to my methods in one of two ways: 1) You'll think I'm an absolute nut-bag and throw this book out your car window while cursing my name with more F-bombs than I dropped the day I found out I was pregnant for the first time (story to follow soon), or 2) You'll say, "Why not?" and choose to trust this process. You must have guts. You must have commitment. You must be tough. You must believe in the big picture. You must feel deep down in your core that keeping yourself organized, practical, and fighting-the-good-fight for focus every day will benefit your child, your spouse, and your own inner strength and confidence in the most unexpected and incredible ways. But it's *your* choice. You must remember this no matter what kind of baby you get.

Lucky for all of us, I've included some perky fab tips throughout this book—enclosed in colored boxes and throughout the body of the text—full of advice and insight from some of my most savvy, smart, and certified experts and famous friends (all mothers, and one dad) who I continue to draw guidance from—you might recognize and be fans of some of them from television and online. I'm not a fitness specialist. These friends of mine agree with me on many things I present in this book, yet also disagree with me about some of my ideas, too. But we all respect each other. (That's the magical thing about motherhood—you learn to respect others' choices quickly . . .)

I'm not a medical doctor. I'm not a shrink. I don't claim to have every impeccable answer for each microscopic circumstance that comes up in a new mom's life—nor do I have faith in anyone who claims they do. A one-size-fits-all solution for anything related to having a baby does not exist. But I am a mother, daughter, wife, sister, and your most sincere, fast talking, no-nonsense, cut-to-the-chase-and-just-do-it friend. Sometimes, I might get bossy. Why? Because finding and keeping your FAB self turned on and pumped up from delivery day through the first year of motherhood and beyond is worth it to yourself and your family for the rest of your life.

No, I will not be encouraging you to neglect your child while you navigate these methods of mine. Rather, your darlings will be driving this mission—just as my daughters steered my discovery for this wacky way of living as a new mom. Contrary to feeling like I lost myself after baby, as so many women struggle with, I *found* myself in the most positive and profound way within the first year of each of my daughters' births. I don't believe I'm alone in figuring out how to bounce back (and I'm certainly not the only one to do it), but I believe this topic is underdiscussed, underrated, and often regarded as undoable in today's parenting community. Here's a fact I've always believed: any woman can bounce back fast after having a baby, including YOU (which is why I wrote this book).

It's go time!

PART 1
WHY BOUNCE BACK?

"Being a mom makes you better. May the force be with you. Go for it."
—Rachel Zoe, mom, fashion designer & celebrity stylist (March 2015)

Who really cares about bouncing back anyway? Isn't a new mom supposed to just relax and relish her new role as a mother while cuddling her new bundle on the couch in the same robe she slept in? Bouncing back fast after babies is only for celebrities with money and access to constant hired help and a Hollywood-driven responsibility to shock and awe us all by strutting in a swimsuit on the cover of *US Weekly* just weeks after childbirth. Much of that is true, yes, but the true benefit for bouncing back fast for us regular chicks has less to do with showing off to our friends and family (although that can certainly be entertaining) and more to do with developing solid resilience to carry us through the trials and triumphs of new motherhood. Bouncing back fast isn't just for Beyoncé; it's for all of us regular superstars, too.

CHAPTER 1
FACTS & FEELINGS

You planned for a baby. You didn't plan for a baby. You had challenges conceiving. It happened faster than you thought it ever would.

No two pregnancies are alike, and they never will be. Every mom's got her own feelings about the hows, whys, and whats of her own life. To bounce back, you must first accept and own what you feel, whatever that feeling is. For me, my obsessive mission described in this book was fueled by a chaotic clash of freaked out identity change and my desperate wish to continue to work on television. (How shallow and confusing, I know.) However, that conflict proved to set the scene for uncovering a most realistic journey about how to become a better woman after baby . . .

The Bumpy Backstory . . .

"You'd better f—ing get in here RIGHT NOW!" I yelled violently to my husband in the other room. Classy, right? It was January 17, 2010. (Man, how I cringe when I think of these words now.)

To my lingering shame, that is what I screamed in the hallway to break the news to my husband that I was pregnant for the first time. I was barefoot in my underwear, in our apartment's small white bathroom, with more tears running down my face than I'd ever cried in my life. The snot was dripping. I'm pretty sure I was shaking. I was inconsolable and remember my heartbeat racing and my body feeling like it was burning hot. I think it was some kind of pregnancy panic attack. My husband ran in, saw the pink plus sign on the counter and my puffy red face. He smiled and said, "It's okay . . . going to be fun." He gave me kiss. I didn't return the kiss but kept crying.

Yes, that was stupid of me, but in that moment, I felt like someone had died (that someone was me). We were newlyweds and not yet planning to start a family. Basically, I was some idiot who got really lucky but was too dumb to see it at the time. Those words continue to be one of the biggest regrets of my life, considering how much I crazy-love my daughters and how beyond grateful I am to be a mom. I know better now.

At the time of this panic attack, I was a busy entertainment journalist and television host hustling jobs with a new series about to air on Travel Channel (called *America's Worst Driver*, which lasted about a minute—major points to you if you remember it). I worked about sixty hours per week; days, nights, weekends, whatever. I loved working and busted my butt for it for years to get to the moderate place of success I had achieved. At that time, nobody was putting pregnant women on TV unless they were already famous . . . and I was definitely not famous. For close to seven months of my pregnancy, I sobbed and whined about the end of my young-and-free life and the impending crash-and-burn of my developing career. *I wasn't done with me yet.*

I feared everything in the most immature way. I feared vomiting during pregnancy. I feared packing on a hundred pounds and not losing any of the baby weight afterward. I feared the ongoing leg-spreading scenario of OB/GYN exams. I feared getting the epidural shot in the back when it was time to have the baby. I feared the epidural not working, requiring me to actually *feel* delivering the baby. I feared how in God's name a baby would even be born out of my you-know-where. I feared not ever fitting into any of my sexy, pre-pregnancy clothes years later. I feared losing all my fire, energy, spark, motivation, and drive. I feared I'd be a real idiot when it came to knowing what to even *do* with a baby—prior to my first-born, I'd never even held a baby before . . . never wanted to, frankly.

I also feared continuing my full-time work schedule and entrusting my baby to a nanny or sitter who would spend more time with my child than I would. I feared making the choice to take a break from work to be home with baby and risk not ever working again. I feared that every child and home-related responsibility would fall on me alone, leaving no time for anything else—hey, I'm Armenian-American, and let's just say our heritage's men aren't generally known for changing diapers or cooking a meal of any kind. (Love ya, Honey.) Most of all, I feared the impending reality of focusing on a baby's needs before my own and potentially losing the person I'd worked so hard to become, professionally and personally, before I was ready for it. I just wasn't ready to be a mom.

In defense of my stupid attitude back then, the biggest perception I had about motherhood—from friends, relatives, work associates, media, and wherever else we all get our information—was negative, confused, exhausted, frazzled, and utterly miserable sounding. Maybe it was because I live in the notorious vanity that is Los Angeles? *Oh, your body will never be the same! You'll never sleep again! Say good-bye to your old life! These kids are driving me crazy! I feel so cooped up in Babyland! All I watch on TV these days is* Sesame Street! *So-and-so is sick again! I can't even put a thought together! Someone's always crying here! My husband and I don't even talk to each other anymore because we're so busy taking care of the babies!*

My head was grateful for a healthy and easy pregnancy, but my heart was not catching up—no matter how many adorable baby bump and new mom-related things I did or bought to try and get in the mood. The thought of all the unknowns ahead of me, and how I'd maintain life as my husband and I knew it to be comfortable and fun, freaked me out. To this day, I'm convinced I experienced some kind of mild and undiagnosed "prepartum" depression. (For the record, there is such a thing—look it up, pay attention to your thoughts and feelings, and seek help if you think you might need it.)

Somewhere in my third trimester, my wits hit me over the head with the fear of becoming one of those stereotypical versions of "the overwhelmed new mother": *I'll be damned if I was going to turn into another hot mess new mom.* I suddenly became determined to bounce back from having a baby like no one else I'd known. My own mother even challenged me to do it. "Within three months," she said, "you'll get back to being YOU." I'm not one to argue with my mom, so that was it. But my true fuel for bouncing back fast was to return myself to working TV-host shape and pick up my hustling show business work right where I'd left off. (Little did I know this baby freaking out about would singlehandedly reinvent my career in media for the better . . .)

No whining. No complaining. No frumpy-dump outfits. No freaking out about "I'm so tired." No excuses. Despite how every book and article I'd read flat-out warned and teased about how much a new baby takes a woman down, I was determined to handle it and prove every one of them wrong. And you'd bet I was going to squeeze back into my pre-pregnancy jeans a few months later, too. (I challenge you to find anyone on Earth who doesn't appreciate *that* experience, baby or not.) I'd run an all-in, personal lifestyle experiment on myself to mindfully and healthfully stay focused and get *better after baby*—for mind, body, and spirit. You know, so I could score another random, short-lived show on Travel Channel.

My baby girl was born and I carried on, instantly falling in love with her in the most unexpected ways and chronicling my day-to-day duties and lifestyle while also making tough choices to stay true to my promise. To my own shock, I did bounce back to feeling "fully functioning" within a few months. I even shot a pilot episode for an entertainment news show (that didn't go anywhere) one month postpartum, wearing my pre-pregnancy clothes. The ongoing question from colleagues, friends, family, and the grocery store checkout lady was: *You just had a baby two months ago?!? You don't look like it!* No nanny. No night nurse. No trainer. No stylist. Not even a housekeeper at the time. I had good days, bad days, and pointless days, as any new mom does, but the big picture of my wild plan was *working*.

Just when I was really coasting into motherhood (about eight months in), and was one of two finalists up for a killer job at CNN (a job I didn't get in the end), the whole thing happened again. *Surprise! You're pregnant! And your first child isn't even one year old!*

Bounce this, bitch. So I decided to give up, buy the frumpiest jeans I could find, and fold up shop. I'm kidding! My big bounce-back experiment continued and succeeded against all ridiculous odds for the second time in two years. I was feeling happy. I was feeling organized (now with two babies under the age of two). I was launching a brand-new, unfamiliar digital endeavor called The FAB Mom, and a reinvented career slowly and suddenly started succeeding in unexpected directions.

And that's when I realized I'd done it. I'd bounced back—pretty quickly—after two back-to-back babies. It shocked the heck out of me and felt fabulous. (Still does.) And it will for you, too. How to start? Let's talk about real resilience . . .

The Science of Bouncing Back.

The art and skill of bouncing back is based on resilience. And, resilience is a science. Like, a real science! (We'll get to the wild and wacky tips about how to bounce back soon, but for now, stick with me.) Researchers have studied the phenomenon of what makes someone resilient and have figured out a lot of pretty cool stuff in recent years. (My high school chemistry teacher is cackling somewhere right now, wondering why I wasn't this passionate about chemistry back when I was sixteen.) According to *TIME Magazine*'s June 2015 article "The Science of Bouncing Back" by Mandy Oaklander, as well as the 2012 book *Resilience: The Science of Mastering Life's Greatest Challenges* by Dr. Dennis Charney and Dr. Steven Southwick, there's a growing amount of credible research aimed at pinpointing what makes certain people more resilient to life's changes, challenges, and hiccups. Contrary to what many of us are led to believe, having resilience has very little to do with personality type, but everything to do with consciously developing and conditioning a chemical skill set inside the brain. This skill set pretty much then kicks into overdrive when we're faced with stress and enables us to overcome hard times and setbacks.

Yes, you heard me: setbacks. As blessed and wonderful as pregnancy and motherhood are, they can also, at some times, bring setbacks. Changes in daily routine, family life, career, time management, relationships—they all count as possible impending setbacks. These holdups are the things that trigger new moms' heads to spin. I've known well-educated and accomplished professionals who lost all sense of how to live everyday life with babies without feeling like a wreck (and then found it again, but years later). I've known women who've always wanted to be stay at home moms question why they're not happy living their dream when, in fact, they're doing exactly what they always wanted to do.

A former television host and strong as you-know-what adventure-junkie friend of mine who once climbed Mount Kilimanjaro will unabashedly tell you that motherhood brought her to her knees—mentally, physically, and emotionally. The reality of pregnancy, birth, and becoming a mother can interrupt our emotions, relationships, workflow, confidence, and day-to-day ability to get things done. See? And as we all know, interruptions and change in our lives as we know them can feel stressful . . . babies included. (Apologies to babies around the world, but it's true.)

One of the most fascinating findings to come from research on bouncing back (at the time of this writing) suggests that we regular folks can actually train ourselves to be more resilient. Research has also found that stress can weaken our resilience. Combine the common and frequent new-mom struggle of major life change, larger-than-life responsibility, hormone readjustment, and sleep deprivation with all the deep complications of regular life (relationships, finances, changing careers, the demands of our oversaturated digital world, and on and on) and no wonder modern parents are extraparanoid when a new baby is born! The digital age has brought tons of information to the fingertips of new moms, but it's also manipulating our ability to let go and making us micromanage our lives as parents. The struggle is real and can cause major stress (even if we're thrilled about having a new baby).

So how do we combat these hectic changes connected with getting over that proverbial bump of new motherhood? We commit to conditioning ourselves throughout pregnancy and the first year according to what modern science has discovered about resilience. I'll spare you the intricate studies and details, but to put it bluntly: it's believed, and some would say been proven, that anyone can develop resilience. By doing certain activities that induce blood flow and natural biochemical production, you can actually train your brain to respond to pressure in a significantly more manageable way, which then improves your quality of life. What new mother doesn't want a better quality of life for herself, her child, and her whole family? There is no one-size-fits-all remedy to boost resilience skills, but ways to foster resilience development do exist.

How to kick-start your brain into learning how to bounce back? Scientists have found the following techniques effective:

- ☺ *Facing things that scare you.* (Tackle your fears!)
- ☺ *Developing a guide for daily decisions.* (Organize your day!)
- ☺ *Building a strong network of social support.* (Find fun friends!)

- ☺ *Making physical exercise a habit.* (Work your body? Better your brain!)
- ☺ *Developing mindfulness.* (Learn to stay in the moment and concentrate on *what* you're doing *when* you're doing it. In other words, make yourself focus! How FAB is that?)

Good thing this book spills all sorts of tricks to get you on track doing what's described above. Becoming a mom is a major life change. The more you are aware of this reality—notice I said *aware of* and not *scared*—the more prepared you will be for the challenges new motherhood presents and the better you will be able to navigate your new life confidently and effectively. For me, the key to regaining focus postbirth was making a choice to mentally get ahead of the impending doom (for lack of a better word). I didn't want to wait for motherhood to tackle and take me down from behind. I was intent about facing my new life with fearless confidence and a conscious choice to be strong in spirit. Choosing to be resilient, no matter what that adorable, screaming, constantly pooping baby throws your way, sets the foundation for a bounce like no other.

Like I said in my introduction: any woman can bounce back after having a baby. Look out, celebrity moms—turns out we're just like *you* now. So where to go from here? Up.

Boost Yourself Up for the Better.

Now that we're smart about the facts for developing resilience, our next order of business is to get our heads in the game. After my own experiments, this is what I know to be true and beneficial for jump-starting this most mind-blowing process: new moms must get a big ego as quickly as possible. You heard me: we must boost ourselves up. Boost ourselves up to think . . . what? Here are my top three thoughts to remember and revisit while tackling all the tips I suggest throughout this book:

- ☺ *We are just like our moms who raised us, but better—we're equipped with the Internet.*
- ☺ *We are the newly hired CEO of a powerful corporation—our babies are our new job, and we will conquer because we actually made them with our own bodies.*
- ☺ *We are capable of doing anything free of judgment—because moms have extra moxie without even trying.*

Think of boosting yourself up as an exercise in mental conditioning: all you're doing is giving yourself daily doses of reassurance and free confidence. When your spouse is at work, your parents live hundreds of miles away, your friends are carting their own kids back and forth (or going about their single, child-free lives), and you're home alone with a brand new baby and having an exceptionally lonely day, you need to know how to pep-talk yourself out of a rut no matter what. Psychologists say it takes anywhere between a few weeks to several months to form a habit, so why not start practicing your own ego-boosting skills while pregnant? The mind will start believing things you tell it, if you tell it the same things frequently and often. *I am smarter than everyone else. I am sexy. Oh yeah.*

Seriously, though, let's start with the part about being just like our moms, but better. True, I most likely don't know your mom, but I have confidence she was fabulous in some way or another. What was it like to be a mother when our moms became new parents? Well, chances are your mom did not have the Internet to consult for every single cut and scrape and cough and sneeze . . . and she survived quite fine and raised you. Growing up, you most likely never doubted that she knew exactly what she was doing (at least that's how I felt as a kid). My mom raised me in an era rampant with cigarette-smoking pregnancies (which she did not do nor do I condone on any level, for the record), open-range parenting practices that included allowing children to walk to and from the school bus stop by ourselves and ongoing phrases like *Go outside and play* as opposed to today's go-to *Let me do that for you, honey*. Past generations of parents also exclusively formula-fed their babies and toted kids across town without car seats. I bet you once rode your bike around the neighborhood without an adult trailing you. If you didn't, you should try it now. It's amazing.

By most personal accounts found online and in my own circle of family and friends, parenting in previous generations was absolutely less stressful than it is today. Hey, I'm not suggesting anyone bust out the ciggies with a bump in tow, but take a look around and notice how high-maintenance and exhausting modern pregnancy and parenting has now become. We question, panic about, and run to Google to research every little thing. There are too many options, and we've got more accessible information and education than we know what to do with. *Which stroller is best? Which birth method is best? What's the best device to strap onto our belly so our unborn child can listen to classical music and be born brilliant? If I don't enroll in a birthing class that's offered by the instructor that's famous around town, will my child be born in the right way?* Our parents raised us without all of today's excess of gear, tools, and online paranoia—and we turned out damn good. Damn good.

It's time to stop questioning and overthinking, and just *do*! For whatever reason, we modern moms (me included) have fooled ourselves into thinking that we must micromanage every single detail of our child's existence. I caught myself doing it as a new mom and still catch myself doing it. *Did she drink enough milk? Why did she only burp once this time? Was that apple organic enough? Did my daughter poop enough today or should I worry?*

Scroll any given mom group on Facebook and you will see never-ending questions and concerns about every single detail of children's existences. It's borderline pathetic how much we can overthink things, and this dangerous cycle often starts during pregnancy. The owner of one of my favorite and longtime neighborhood shops for pregnant and new moms told me how so many of her most recent customers and clients seem to be irrationally fearful of everything—and how frustrating and counterproductive it is for new motherhood. Paying attention and being concerned about our baby's well-being is smart (and recommended), but being paranoid and losing all common sense—common sense that we once had prebaby—is not.

Resist falling into the trap of micromanaged parenting and start boosting your own rational thoughts during pregnancy as soon as you can: *Life is good. Pregnancy is merely pregnancy. All is fine. All will be fine. My mom did this and so will I. No problem, because I'm capable. My grandmother had to hand-wash dishes, clothes, and diapers and she figured out how to make it all work. Babies in Africa poop on the dirt and they live perfectly happy lives. I'm not the first woman in the world to have a baby, so stop acting like it.* Moms of the past were women who got pregnant, had babies, and raised children. Moms of today are also women who get pregnant, have babies, and raise children. Previous generations raised smart, kind people without all the drama that modern new motherhood has become, and so can we. The fact that we're better equipped with technology and information is icing on the cake—not to be abused and get confused by. You. Can. Handle. It. So handle it. You get me?

Moving on to our next boosting point: remind yourself that you're about to be (or have just been) promoted to CEO of a powerful company. (Some people I know like to say CMO, Chief Mom Officer—you say whatever floats your boat.) That's right, think of your new and growing family as a corporation with you as the leader. This corporation has big expectations. It's all hands on deck, and you've got to bungee off that cliff and hit that deck running to keep your job and get that bonus at the end of the year.

As a new mom, your job is to stay rational, hustle your vision, problem-solve with quick smarts, and provide confident leadership so everyone you work with can do their jobs effectively. No excuses. No turning back. No doubting your capability. They hired *you* . . . and you're perfect for the job. You won't let them down simply because you've already done a heck of a lot in your life and you know how to get things done (more about how to jog your own memory and make past accomplishments relevant in your new-mom life later). I'll bet the smart and capable prebaby you would rise to the occasion to succeed at a new job—so must the new-mom you.

Recognizing yourself as a leader sets a fine scene for our final point: truly believing that you can do almost anything free of judgment. (No one questions the boss.) My first taste of telling myself to believe I could do anything "just because I was a soon-to-be CMO" came during my ninth month of my first pregnancy. It was equal parts powerful and pathetic; I forced my way into an audition for a brand new television show, to be considered as the host, with a baby bump sticking out to kingdom come.

Long story short, I had a previously booked audition that was soon canceled by the show's executive producers at the last minute. It was never said outright, but all evidence of events pointed to the cause for cancellation as being my big belly and impending birth. My agent at the time gave the producer a heads-up that I was nine months with child ahead of my meeting, and then—*poof!*—they were suddenly not interested to meet me. Yes, I was expecting to deliver a baby very soon and production was to start one week after my due date, but I was livid about being told that I could not interview for a job because of a baby bump. (In case you're curious, the show I'm talking about here was SyFy network's award-winning movie makeup artist challenge *Face Off*.)

I made phone calls to friends of friends who knew the production team and connected me to them directly so I could convince the boss to see me for an audition despite his abrupt cancellation. *I could go to the audition anyway and blow them away and change their minds and push the entire production schedule back a few months on account of my talent and charisma!* (I was hormonally delusional.) I wore my lowest-cut, loosest-fitting top to simultaneously show off my amazing cleavage and minimize my belly (again, delusional). I'd told myself enough times that I belonged at that audition no matter what near-birth state I was in, so I started believing it. My agent tried to talk me out of this stunt, but I didn't listen. I am now positive the producer thought I was nuts and only agreed to see me for the purpose of preventing a lawsuit citing maternal discrimination from a crazy lady.

I stomped into that meeting with full hair, makeup, bigger boobs than I'd ever had in my life, high heels, tight maternity jeans, and an out-of-this world perky attitude. I read the script a few times, and we had a laugh about how I was genuinely ready to pop out a baby any second. I may've made an ass of myself, but I was shocked at how I felt afterward: I was higher than a kite. It was one of my best auditions ever (minus the conversation about my water potentially breaking on camera).

Why did it feel so good? It had everything to do with total belief in myself and not a shred of doubt for my actions. *Aha! This is the grade of confidence required to jump-start motherhood. With focused persistence like this, I can overcome any kind challenge a newborn chucks at me, no problem.* (I didn't get the job. Hello, they were starting a hundreds-of-thousands-of-dollars production one week after my due date. *I* wouldn't have given me that job. I now know the executive producer personally, and we've laughed about this stunt of mine since.)

If you boost yourself into believing something, you actually do start believing it, and "it" becomes reality. You're just like the mom who raised you, except better equipped, which makes you exponentially capable of all kinds of amazing if you keep rationality in check. You're the new CMO and can truly do anything, because they hired *you* for the job. Plant those thoughts in your head, memorize and believe them, write them down to read the day after delivery, and then post them to your fridge and bathroom mirror so you see them every day. Make a habit to boost yourself up for the better. You are the boss who can handle anything, even a newborn baby.

Time to talk bumps!

PART 2
THE BUMPY MONTHS
OF PREPARATION

"Hormones, mood swings, and crying mascara down my face is definitely not fab. Passing out at 9 p.m. at the dinner table or an event [because I'm so tired] is not so fab either. During pregnancy, you need to do whatever you can to make yourself feel good and look good. So for me, that means wearing heels and getting dressed up . . ."
—Anya Sarre, mom, celebrity stylist & television personality (May 2012)

Here's the big secret that you may or may not want to hear: bouncing back after baby truly begins *during* the third trimester of pregnancy. Taking advantage of the last months the baby is still in your belly to gear up your mind, get in tune with your body, and boost your spirit is just good planning. In other words: get organized before you have a kid to take care of, before your days and nights get confused. If you're pregnant while reading this and on your way, excellent! If not, don't fret. You can skim this section for kicks, giggles, and future reference and then hit things hard the next time around. Let's start with the body . . .

CHAPTER 2

PREPARING YOUR BODY FOR THE BOUNCE

I'm going to take a guess that when you saw the cover of this book, you thought, *This is going to teach me to get my body back!* Am I right? Sorry if you're disappointed about the whole "focused and F-A-B" acronym thing, but you make a good point—most people think *body* when the concept of bouncing back after baby is brought up: how to dress, how to look good, how to get the baby weight to melt away with only a smidge of effort. (I hear you there.) So, we'll give you the thing you may've bought and opened this book for first . . .

Use Your Boobs & Wear . . . Black?

Yes, you read that correctly. "Use. Your. Boobs." (How sexist.) Hey, bosoms get bigger with pregnancy. For small-chested women like me, suddenly having knockers was one of my most favorite perks, which I shamelessly showed off, without apology, through my pregnancy. (Is this sexist?) I'm not going to lie and tell you that I didn't enjoy having cleavage for the first time in my life, because I did. (Is this even appropriate that I'm putting this in print?) Looking down at my chest in a low-cut top made me feel sexy on my most unsexy-feeling days. That's that naked truth. Looking in the mirror and seeing real cleavage, as opposed to the kind that flat-chested girls like me shadow in with bronzer and a makeup brush, made me giddy. It was fun. It was funny. Every expecting mom needs as much fun and funny as she can hijack.

Near the end, I turned my questionable and immature behavior into a game. *How far can I unbutton my blouse before my husband says something like, "Are you really going to go out like that?"* We're all grown-ups here. Live it up, ladies. Wear the low-cut tops. Enjoy the extra curves. I mean, we see how celebrities do it up these days—not much is shocking to anyone anymore when it comes to pregnancy style. If Kim Kardashian West gets away with that totally sheer black lace sheath that revealed her belly on the red carpet a few years ago, no one's going to give your low-cut top a second look. Actresses Kerri Washington and Blake Lively are famous for their maternity dresses with cutouts and belly-revealing slits and crops. Kinda risky, but they did it anyway. Don't be shy, embarrassed, or take yourself too seriously unless you're going to church or work or a PTA meeting or something—then absolutely cover it up.

You want a deeper, more meaningful reason to amp up the cookies? Fine, here's my personal take: showing off the goods builds confidence with your body and develops your resilience on a mental level to not be intimidated by how you think others might view you—not in an "in your face" way, but in a "Hey, this is my body and I'm going to own it" way . . . for yourself. (Trust me, there will be plenty of judgment about how you choose to dress and parent once that baby comes.) To drive this argument home, I'll take us back to what was known online as #Cleavage-Gate in early 2016, when Oscar-winning actress Susan Sarandon got major flak from television pundit Piers Morgan for showing off ample cleavage at the age of sixty-nine. No, Ms. Sarandon was not expecting a child, but whether you thought it was fabulous or offensive, this much is true: it takes a confident broad to pull off something like that. (The irony of this whole thing is that Susan's daughter, Eva Amurri, is now an insanely popular mom on Instagram—her site is HappilyEvaAfter.com.)

Take a few opportunities during pregnancy to build confidence about your changing body, not for the sake of making others uncomfortable or shocking the world on Instagram, but for the sake of feeling secure no matter what look you look like. Making an effort to get comfortable with your body, and all its unfamiliar pregnancy shapes and changing sizes, will covertly prompt you to tackle new motherhood head-on without intimidation, apology, or uncertainty once it's time to take care of a baby. Those who are confident in their own skin tend to be more comfortable with making decisions, whether those choices are about what to eat for lunch, which guidelines to follow when introducing solid foods to your child, or which color to paint the nursery.

Once the baby comes, your breasts will do all sorts of crazy stuff, and the supple magic will be gone just like that. What if your boobs are out of control and driving you nuts? Keep everything supported with a proven and sturdy maternity bra. This too shall pass. Now that's all I'm going to say about this, because how much can you really write about making the most of your pregnancy ta-tas without sounding like a sexist or seriously disturbed person? Not much. (Time's up.)

As for wearing black, this was just a lazy trick I came up with during my own experiences. I've been pregnant in summer and winter, and wearing black during both seasons made me feel sexy regardless of how big and uncomfortable my belly got. Wearing black is slimming, timeless, and looks organized no matter what kind of pants, skirt, dress, or blouse combo you might throw together.

You can imagine how much I felt like a smarty-pants when celebrity stylist and designer Rachel Zoe shared her biggest postpartum fashion tip with me at her maternity clothing line launch in 2015: "More black." She said, "I have two [baby] boys that are constantly eating and basically what happens is that I'm holding them, I'm on the ground, and all I take is a baby wipe and go 'zshink' and I wipe it off and that's it." Enough said, I think. Don't question whether you look like you're attending a funeral—just accept that you're going to look sleek and that's the end of the story.

Another trick I used toward the end of my pregnancies was opting to wear a very limited wardrobe. What were the five most useful pieces I wore over and over? Leggings, tank tops, a long and open sweater that covered my butt (the same kind of pieces we saw Kim Kardashian West flaunting everywhere during her most recent pregnancy), a puffy wraparound scarf to draw attention away from my belly, and floor-length dresses to make me look and feel like some kind of goddess-mother-in-the-making. I also wore lots of wedged heels because I couldn't bear to part with the false height I'd gotten myself accustomed to during my twenties.

(Fine, I did get one pair of flats to wear toward the end for safety purposes only . . . I give you permission, too.)

My real reason for wearing a restricted, all-black wardrobe was this: it made my life easier. The less energy I spent thinking about "What the hell can I put on today that will look fab, when I don't feel so fab," the better my day was. The less time wasted pulling on that billowy purple maternity blouse I bought in an effort to look festive, just to take it off again because I felt like I was channeling Barney the Dinosaur with a belly, the more time there was to focus on preparing myself and my home for the forthcoming baby. See my point? Don't waste any time, anywhere. Streamlining options—even if it's only about what you wear—makes life more manageable and enjoyable. Mastering this small step of knowing how to eradicate wasted time will add up after your baby arrives, and learning how to shave time where you can is absolutely important for bouncing back. Trust me.

3 Fixes for Dressing the Bump Fabulously

From Anya Sarre, mom, celebrity stylist, TV style expert

I first met Anya at a celebrity event when she was around seven months pregnant; she was decked in a knockout maxidress, glitzy designer heels, and hair and makeup that would make any A-list star envious while interviewing pregnant celebrities on the red carpet. I was fascinated with how fabulous she looked and how *friendly* she was one-on-one. We got to know each other a bit, and, every time I see her on television, either styling someone or dishing about the best must-have fashion and beauty products, I listen up good.

31

1. **Accessories are your best friend**. If you have never been a fan of accessories, now is your chance! Dress up your bump with long, layered necklaces, statement earrings, or stacked bangle bracelets. Accessories draw the eye away from your bump to keep your head-to-toe look streamlined and proportioned.

2. **Don't fight your changing body, smooth it . . .** No one tells you that a perfectly round bump does not appear overnight. Shapewear can be the magic trick to a smooth, sleek silhouette. I know what you're thinking—shapewear is uncomfortable and will make you sweaty, but not always. The best maternity shapewear I've found is Pea in the Pod's stretch biker shorts. They feel like pajamas, and you might still wear them after your bump is gone.

3. **Bet on your bra!** Pregnancy and new motherhood often call for new bras, so make sure you find one that is super-comfortable, fashionable, and can add a layer to your wardrobe. My favorite secret is the Coobie Seamless Bra—it gives a no-bulge, seamless look under any outfit (no back-fat!), is one-size-fits-all, and can fit you through an entire pregnancy. Women have been known to sleep, work out, and go out in them. You can even layer a Coobie lace design with a longer tank (and shorter tank over it) to give the bump a smooth, styled look.

Take Care of the Belly.

Pay attention to these three words: Vitamin E Oil. Sure, you can use modern creams, new-age elasticity potions, and a classic bottle of cocoa butter (man I do love the smell . . . it's like you're on vacation), but old-school and inexpensive Vitamin E Oil from the drugstore can also minimize (and in my case, totally prevent) the appearance of stretch marks like a real mother. You can credit my former makeup artist Francine from my entertainment news days for this one. (Hi, Frannie!)

Years before I got married and became pregnant, Francine and I had one of those out-of-nowhere conversations that you only have with people you're really close to, or who see you at your absolute worst to do your hair and makeup and make you feel beautiful and powerful every single day for three and a half years straight. For some reason, I was spilling my guts about how inexplicably petrified I was about a far-off future pregnancy: giving birth, how the body handles it, what would happen to my career, and on and on (I think she may've been putting false eyelashes on me at the time). Francine was kind, cool, had two little girls of her own—and an insanely rockin' body.

One day she offered me the most valuable advice for pregnancy that I credit for kick-starting my bounce back the first time around: "If you rub Vitamin E Oil all over, on your boobs, stomach, butt, and upper arms from the very beginning, it helps your skin a lot." Who was I to question a longtime Hollywood makeup artist who'd made some of media's most popular television celebrities beautiful over the course of her career? I remember sitting in the chair thinking, *I will remember this for when it's time.* Sure enough, I remembered her wisdom years later when that infamous pink plus sign showed up and I dropped that shameful F-bomb of mine in my bathroom. That same day, I went to the store (with my face still red and puffy from crying to my husband) and bought prenatal vitamins and the biggest bottle of generic bright-yellow Vitamin E Oil on the bottom shelf. From finding out I was five weeks pregnant up until the birth of my babe, I slathered on that magic potion two to three times a day on my boobs, belly, butt, legs, and arms. *If Francine said this works, then it must work.*

My ritual was once in the morning, once midday, and once before bed. Sometimes, I'd mix things up and replace the midday rubdown with cocoa butter just to give my skin a break from all the oil (and to smell that yummy tropical scent). Skin and beauty experts continuously suggest: the trick for minimizing stretch marks is to start *early* in pregnancy with the moisturizing to get ahead of the skin-stretching process as a belly grows, rather than waiting until the belly has already popped. I greased up for nine straight months. You could've fried me like a potato.

Lubing up the belly is big news and big business these days, as I'm sure you're aware. As I later found out, actress, television personality, and gorgeous mom of three Ali Landry and I shared similar rituals. She told me during an interview a few years back, "I lathered my body twenty-four hours a day in Palmer's Cocoa Butter. The key is to stay lathered up all over your body, as much as you can . . . I also drank a ton of water." (It should be noted that Landry did serve as a paid spokesperson for Palmer's. But, paid spokesperson or not, it worked for her.)

Did I have stretch marks after my first baby arrived? Nope. My second pregnancy around, I practiced the same ritual and ended up having a few pale marks that faded over time. Was it all dumb luck? It certainly could've been. The hard truth is that skin condition and elasticity is mostly genetic—ask any dermatologist. No preventative remedy is 100-percent effective for everyone across the board, thanks to all of us being different with our own DNA. But oiling up obsessively yielded almost unbelievable results for *me*. Why not try it for you? Experiment with the innovative and expensive creams or try plain Vitamin E Oil if you like to save a buck. Whatever you choose to do, do it consistently.

In addition to rubbing down your belly, it's also a good idea to intentionally *respect* the bump and *own* it—not in a weird hippy-dippy kind of way, but in a most level-headed, wow-there-is-a-person-in-here kind of way. One of my biggest fails from my first time around was that it took me a shameful amount of time to positively regard my pregnancy for the fun and funny miracle it was. I wasted so much time feeling frustrated about my clothes no longer fitting and wondering when it'd all be over and I could get on with life. I refused to even consider doing one of those trendy, bump-centric photo shoots because I was convinced I'd never want to see any kind of image of me being pregnant after in future years (I was wrong). It took actress and big-screen sex symbol Eva Mendes to turn my head right.

I was almost eight months pregnant and was assigned to interview Eva for her new movie at the time. I wore a dark purple, sleeveless A-line dress that loosely draped over my bump with super-high heels. The dress was also really low cut, which boosted the fun factor a bit (heed the "use your boobs" section). Despite the cleavage factor, my belly was getting on my nerves big time, as so many women relate to as the end of pregnancy nears. All I could think the morning of our interview, as I was getting ready in my bathroom, was *Crap, this bump is out of control. How am I going to physically climb up into that tall director chair across from her and not look ridiculous or be distracting? She'll probably wonder why I'm there bothering with the effort in the first place.* I felt embarrassed for feeling the pressure to be sexy, savvy, and smart on camera across from a huge Hollywood celebrity this late in the pregnancy game (remember, back then, pregnancy wasn't a "cool" thing seen on television frequently like it is now). Maybe she would be distracted by my shoes—my heels were smokin' and really high.

I remember waddling in to the interview and smiling really big in an effort to keep her eyes on my face rather than my bump. To my stunned shock, Eva made a big deal of how "adorable!" my bump was the second I walked in. She stood up and offered to help me climb into the chair. "Oh my gosh! How are you feeling? You are adorable! I hope I look like you when it's my turn!" *Say what woman? Um, I'd like to look like you right now, Eva.*

I'd interviewed Eva a few times in previous years, but by no means did we have any kind of personal friendship or special affection for each other—I doubt she recognized me from the times we'd met at all. I was a journalist doing my job, she was a movie star doing hers. But her immediate respect and joy for my midsection watermelon caught me off guard, as this was years before she became a mother herself. There she was, unintentionally making me realize what a jerk I'd been acting like and prompting me to respect my own bump. *Shame on me.*

My mind shifted right then and there. (Acceptance is a powerful thing.) From that day, I started making efforts to "take care of my bump," which set me up for more practical and physical comfort before and after baby. If the belly's giving you pain, challenge yourself to do something about it—opt to stay home and rest if you don't feel like going to that party, keep your body supported by wearing one of the dozens of pregnancy-slings you can buy at practically any maternity store, experiment with keeping your belly propped up at night (by lying sideways) with one of those long body pillows to increase your comfort and chances of getting more sleep. Curb the complaining and start *solving and doing*. If you've got an ailment driving you batty, I guarantee there's a contraption or latest technique that just might solve some of your issues—find what you need as soon as you feel like you might need it.

One of the keys to bouncing back after baby is knowing how to actively and immediately problem-solve a situation and not complain to the point that it drags you down. Start getting into the habit of helping yourself quickly and efficiently as soon as you need it, rather than just feeling helpless and uncertain, before the baby comes along. You can vent, but vent and then be done with it so you can bounce along. You know yourself best, so don't be lazy about paying attention and helping yourself when you need it. It's not vanity; it's biology. Which leads me to . . .

Watch Your Butt.

Loaded Topic Alert here. As we all know, the issue of weight—before, during, and after babies and birth—is a spicy topic that can send even the most level-headed women into incendiary fights and arguments we can't come back from. (You'll see.) This section is all about being aware and responsible about weight gain during pregnancy. There. I said it.

Please keep in mind this is one of the most delicate yet tougher-talking parts of this book, and by no means is it intended to be any kind of a shaming, berating, or condescending conversation that picks apart weight gain during pregnancy. *Hello! Weight gain is normal, mandatory, and absolutely expected and welcome for pregnancy!* However, this conversation is about being conscious of choices involving food and exercise during pregnancy. My doctor will tell you that I gained a healthy amount of weight during pregnancy both times around. But what I'm about to humbly share with you comes from a most honest place, in the name of giving you *power and perspective.* This is a safe space. I am your friend. If you want the satisfaction of what it feels like to bounce back fast from the inside-out, have faith that getting your body back as much as possible after delivery *is a part of the whole experience* to serve you well mentally, physically, and spiritually after baby.

Before we get into the nitty-gritty, I'll share a true story that fires me up every time I think about it (just so you know where I'm coming from about this): One of my first interactions with someone, outside of my family and immediate friends, about post-baby bodies, went something like this: "You bitch, you've already lost your baby weight." I had no idea how to react. It was a few months after my delivery, I was out with friends for the first time and feeling pretty good about myself until her comment shattered me.

Yes, this woman was trying to be funny and snarky . . . but what she said put me on major defense and made me feel superuncomfortable, ashamed, and guilty. *Why should I feel guilty for looking like myself after baby?* I then started thinking about how and why I'd managed to return to my prebaby self so "quickly," as she accused me of, and came up with this: bouncing back my body after pregnancy was easier because a) I was in shape before getting knocked up and b) I was mindful about pregnancy weight gain.

The brutal bottom line here: the more fit you are before pregnancy, and the less empty weight you gain during pregnancy, the more agile you will be with less extra weight on your body after birth. (Again, I ask that that statement not be twisted to mean that a woman should diet or not gain weight during pregnancy.) Dealing with the emotional roller coaster of changing physicality, while fighting sleep deprivation and managing all that goes with a newborn, is extremely personal, sensitive, and complicated beyond discussion. However, making an effort to be responsible with pregnancy weight gain is something everyone can do *at their own pace*. We all know pregnancy prompts weird things to happen in the body; hormone surges, water retention, and stress can make expecting women gain weight beyond all logic. Some weight gain is controllable, some isn't. Don't worry about things you can't control like water retention and hormone spikes, but opt to control your own effort when it comes to food and exercise during pregnancy.

Putting effort into something, when so much is out of your control and you don't know if it will work at all or not, is always scary (especially since results are not guaranteed), but let's recall our earlier chat about training yourself for resilience near the beginning of this journey: *Resilience muscles can be trained by facing things that scare you* . . . The more your resilience skill set is trained during pregnancy—food choices and exercise included—the more your brain will be "trained" for resilience, and the better you'll be able to problem solve clearly and cope with stress tied to crying, colicky, fussy, nonsleepy, unpredictable, and hungry babies in the near future. (Gotcha there, didn't I?)

So here's one of the wacked-out things that proved worthy for me during my pregnancies: I looked to new celebrity moms for inspiration rather than deflation. My first time around, I read stories about Bethenny Frankel's yoga sessions, Giselle Bundchen's postpartum bikini photoshoots, and how supermom Brooke Burke-Charvet pretty much wore her "regular jeans" throughout her pregnancy. True, celebrities are blessed with rare and incredible genetic codes that can be downright annoying to look at, but make an effort to spin everything you see about celebrity moms into a positive perspective for you to mimic at your own pace . . . because, why not?

You want an example? Fine. When I was about six weeks into my first pregnancy, I remember watching some random video interview online that featured Brooke Burke-Charvet talking about how she kept her butt and legs fit enough to wear her pre-pregnancy jeans for as long as possible by just unbuttoning the top button and unzipping the zipper. . . . I figured I could try that, too. (I pulled it off up to month six. See? Possible.) I didn't kill myself exercising; I just made an effort to gently keep up my workouts and moderately continue to work my legs and butt to keep them intact as my belly grew bigger. It worked, great. If it didn't, then so what? I'd just try for the heck of it.

Celebrities may have resources the rest of us can't really tap into, but they're still just people. I say this because I've talked to literally hundreds of them up close and personal in sit-down interviews and on red carpets. Some of these goddesses have bumpy skin. Some of them have cellulite. Some of them have more hair extensions that you'd never second-guess at first glance—and don't forget the false eyelashes, too. I'm also obligated to remind you that most all those pictures we see have been airbrushed and shaved and altered beyond what you might imagine rational—chances are that celebrity mom's postbaby midsection feels a hell of a lot squishier than it looks in the photo and might just resemble us more in real life than we're led to believe. Keeping this reality is mind while scrolling actress and dancer Jenna Dewan Tatum's racy Instagram feed of her killer abs in bikinis and leotards postbaby softens the blow, no? (No, I'm not drunk as I write this.)

But what about Blake Lively getting into a tiny bikini for that movie in the ocean just months after having a baby? There's no way you can airbrush that kind of stuff on film! Yes, Blake also reportedly exercised six days a week with an intense trainer to make it all happen—because she was contractually bound to make it happen and her big fat paycheck and a multimillion-dollar production depended on her to pull it off. Celebrities are regular people with lots of thanks to high-stakes career requirements. And, let's not forget that Blake was beyond physically fit before pregnancy, too.

Set your goal as this: aim to pull off a "mini, realistic version" of what many celebrity moms pull off after having babies, minus airbrushing, personal trainers, and posh delivered meals prepared by one of those chefs that work for Oprah. We buy bargain versions of celebrity clothes so we can set ourselves up to be "bargain versions" of their postbaby personas. Challenge yourself to return as close to your actual prebaby body as it was just before getting knocked up within four months after birth. Notice I said your *actual* body before baby—not the fantasy body in your head, not supermodel Gigi Hadid's body, not the body you once had in high school—but your most recent prebaby body that existed the day you saw that positive pregnancy test result. If you weighed 140 pounds before getting pregnant, then your goal is return to 140 pounds after baby no less. And to make it all even more realistic, add 5 to 10 pounds to your expectation, just for good measure (hey, 10 pounds isn't really all that much).

I know what you're thinking: *You bitch. Just because this worked for you doesn't mean it works for all women.* I agree. I also attest to the expert-backed reality that the more fit a body before and during pregnancy, the quicker and better it will bounce back after baby. But that doesn't mean that anyone who didn't have a six-pack before the baby bump is screwed. I can tell you that, based on firsthand experiences across a wide variety of friends—all with different shapes and sizes—who did return to their prebaby bods a few months after giving birth, getting back to your own body within three or four months after delivery has nothing to do with pressure, starvation, excessive exercising, or selfishly neglecting your newborn, but has everything to do with having a healthy respect for your body, a bit of biological fact, and simple math.

As I've said before, I'm not pretending to be a certified fitness expert. I also can't speak to the issue of carrying twins, having to go on bed rest, or having a high-risk pregnancy, but here's what my own ob-gyn told me back in the day, according to approved mainstream medical guidelines at the time: for an average, healthy woman to grow one baby, it is generally recommended that weight gain over a nine-month period hover between 25 and 35 pounds, maybe even up to 40 if the mom was especially petite to begin with. It is not suggested or complacently accepted to gain 50, 60, 70, or even more pounds (as media steers us to believe is okay) just because a woman is expecting. Having an open awareness and conversation about gaining pregnancy weight is not negative or shaming; it's a health issue that should be talked about matter-of-factly, without drama or sensitive feelings involved.

Consider these general facts I stumbled across when thinking about returning to your pre-pregnancy weight:

- *The average weight of a newborn is about 7 to 7.5 pounds*
- *The placenta weighs around 1.5 pounds*
- *Amniotic fluid accounts for approximately 1.8 pounds*
- *The muscle layer of the uterus expands and packs on an extra 2 pounds*

- *Your blood volume increases dramatically during pregnancy and can weigh 2.5 pounds*
- *Extra body fluid, water retention, your boobs, and extra fat storage typically accounts for an extra 12.5 pounds, on average*

Add everything up and you're just under 28 pounds. Throw in a bit more ice cream and French fries for fun and *bam*—you still probably find yourself hovering below the medically recommended pregnancy weight-gain ceiling of 35 pounds, let's say 33 pounds just for math's sake. Subtract the presumed average 7-pound weight of a baby and you're left with about 26 pounds. Once the amniotic fluid and placenta are out (right after delivery of the baby), the water retention starts to wear off, and you finish bleeding down-there after a full week or two, you'll most likely be naturally down another 6 to 8 pounds—10 pounds if you've somehow been blessed by maternity gods. So, in theory, that leaves you with about 16 to 18 real pounds to actually lose. If you set a goal to lose 1 to 2 pounds per week, as is suggested and deemed healthfully possible by experts, you're back in your old clothes by your baby's four-month birthday maybe even his three month birthday. And if you have a larger baby, you're up across the board by a few more pounds. So what.

I know, every body is different, life can go haywire, hormones can be insane and cause tons of weight gain, and weight loss can't be planned on paper like this . . . but I'm just providing generic, science-based averages here so we have something to work from. The baby weight thing doesn't seem so intimidating and dramatic when you break it down like this, now does it? (Now you know: I'm a visual person.) Two weeks after my first daughter's birth, I was down 16 pounds—it was about the same for my second daughter, too. For kicks and giggles, I'll remind us all that Kim Kardashian West did inform her flailing fans via her app that she was down 17 pounds about 11 days after giving birth to her second baby in 2015—that's added incentive for you to know that a sizable amount of baby weight is in fact bodily fluids that just need to expel from your system at their own pace. So, take comfort in that and clap your hands in wild applause for weight loss every time you change a postpartum maxi-pad. (Too graphic?)

Along with resisting shoving fifteen donuts in your mouth within a five-minute period every hour on the hour for the sheer I'm-pregnant-so-what sport of it, light and easy exercise is now officially and widely recommended (by ob-gyns) for an easier birth experience. Moderate exercise is also imperative for a feasible bounceback afterward. Talk to your doctor about what's okay and what's not, but stick with a realistic routine as long as you're safely and physically able. I exercised up until almost the end of month nine for both of my pregnancies—the first time around I pulled off exercising two to three times per week; the second time around my fitness effort only happened about once a week, but I kept going. *Keep going as long as you feel well, even if it's only a walk around the neighborhood once a week. Every little bit adds up.*

Studies have shown that women who exercise during pregnancy regard their bodies more positively than women who don't. Also, exercise does affect our body's ability to birth babies, handle the postpartum physical changes better, and enable us to lose the weight more easily after delivery. During pregnancy, an average woman has close to 50 percent *more* blood in her body and nearly 30 percent more oxygen in her blood—all of which needs to be moved and circulated for widespread health reasons.

Several years ago (before the days of "fit pregnancy experts" that you can now find click after click online), celebrity fitness trainer Tracy Anderson got tons of flak for speaking about how important it is for women to maintain physical fitness during and after pregnancy. She got slammed by a lot of ignorant, loud-mouthed folks on TV just for insisting expecting women stay physical for the sake of conditioning their body's resilience. Everyone thought she was shaming pregnancy weight just because she happens to be a hot-bodied celebrity fitness personality. She wasn't shaming anybody—she was *educating in her own celebrity-inspired way.*

The practical reality about pregnancy fitness is that: the muscle strength you build and maintain during the bump months will come in handy for delivery. The physical stamina you develop will also help you function, day to day, after the baby's born. Tending to a newborn involves sleep-deprived manual labor and rivals some of the most serious boot camps—and you can't succeed at boot camp if you haven't trained for it. Consider your pregnancy fitness effort, as minimal as it might have to be, as boot camp for physical stamina after baby arrives. And if this weren't reason enough, a study by the University of Michigan in early 2016 showed that one quarter of women surveyed experienced stress fractures, thanks to childbirth, similar to the kind of injuries that many endurance athletes experience—41 percent had pelvic muscle tears, two-thirds suffered from severe muscle strain, 15 percent of women suffered from birth injuries that don't quite ever heal. Generally speaking, a physically fit body is more capable of healing itself than an unfit one.

Also, if you recall our scientific explanation about resilience at the beginning of this book, you'll remember that physical exercise automatically sharpens your mentality, which builds lifelong skillsets associated with bouncing back from setbacks more easily. (Yes, looking into the mirror and seeing a reflection that looks nothing like your prebaby self can be a mental setback.) Watch your weight gain rationally and exercise during pregnancy, build muscle strength and memory, look similar to the person you were before the bump, feel good about yourself easily. See what happens here? It's a cyclical process that keeps your morale boosted at a most sensitive and transitional point in the new-mom journey—the part that comes right after birthing a baby. Tracy was right about staying fit through pregnancy; the world outside Hollywood just wasn't ready to admit it.

Turns out, thousands of moms also weren't ready to admit it online in May 2016. Sia Cooper, popular blogger and Instagram fitness queen (@diaryofafitmommy if you want to look her up), got an online lashing for posting pictures of her ripped postbaby bod and rock-hard abs to make any Fitness America contestant jealous about one week after the birth of her second child. The usual accusations went flying like you-know-what hitting a fan: *She bounced back too quickly. She's not healthy. She's not normal. Stop with the unattainable postbaby body!* The fact is, Sia was extremely fit before pregnancy, maintained a doctor-approved workout regimen during pregnancy, and then let her body cash in on the muscle memory she'd built years and years in the making. Don't blame her for laying the groundwork before babies were blips in her mind.

So you want to know my personal stats? Fine. It's only fair for me to share since I'm pushing this most unconventional and blunt philosophy about keeping a hawk-eye on your weight and exercise. (I will preface this whole thing by saying that I was admittedly in great shape before my first pregnancy . . . not like Sia, but admittedly great shape.) Ready? Okay. Weight gained during first pregnancy: 29 pounds. I was able to zip up one pair of my old (looser) jeans five weeks after delivery and fit back into the rest of my old clothes around two months afterward. Weight gained during second pregnancy: 33 pounds. I was back into most of my old clothes somewhere after the three-month mark. I remember being playfully interrogated by the grocery store checkout lady: "Are you sure she's really your baby? You don't *look* like you just had a baby." I always felt like a billion bucks . . . which gave me adrenaline hits every time . . . which gave me added energy to get more things done at home. Offer any new mom surges of energy and she's going to take them without question. (I'll elaborate on fitness specifics that I did implement at home *after* baby later on . . .)

So what can you do? A few of the most popular fitness options for pregnancy:

- ☺ Swimming
- ☺ Yoga
- ☺ Elliptical Machine (as there's very little impact without bouncing)
- ☺ Low-Impact Aerobics
- ☺ Slow Stretching
- ☺ Walking
- ☺ Light/Moderate Weight Training (but only if you weight-trained before!)

What to avoid? Check with your doc, but keep these in mind as not ideal for baby:

- ☺ Any sport that might make you fall

- ☺ Gymnastics
- ☺ Horseback riding
- ☺ Downhill skiing
- ☺ Bungee jumping
- ☺ Rollerblading
- ☺ Contact sports (basketball, soccer)
- ☺ Full sit-ups (These bad boys can cause abdominal muscles to separate or tear from the midline.)
- ☺ Bouncy stretching (Ligaments are already loose during pregnancy—to prepare the body for birth—so don't force a stretch more than what feels moderate.)
- ☺ Hot yoga or excessively hot weather (If a pregnant lady gets too hot, blood gets circulated away from the uterus, and away from baby, to cool the rest of the body off. Not good.)

Keep in mind, if something hurts or feels wrong (you'll know), stop doing it!

My noncertified expert (and doctor-approved) goal was to keep exercising the same way I did prior to expecting a baby, with the exception of running—my doc told me it can sometimes put the uterus at risk of detaching because of the bounciness, but check with your own medical advisor. I kept my favorite activities and just took everything down a notch. I lowered my impact. I reduced my speed. I kept things limited to short spurts, rather than endurance-type rounds. I didn't push things; I merely set out to *maintain* my body parts that didn't involve the bump. I did arm exercises using light weights. I did leg exercises lying on the ground on my back. I did butt exercises on my hands and knees, with my belly almost touching the floor (that was a sight to see and had one particular beefed-up dude looking very confused at my gym). During my third trimesters, I had a thing for taking thirty-minute walks around my neighborhood, doing push-ups against my bathroom sink, and impromptu squats before brushing my teeth at night, but that's what worked for me.

My doctor and I openly discussed my weigh-ins via her office's scale at my standard checkups. I remember one particular appointment had her a bit concerned that I'd gained too much weight too fast, so she asked me to take extra care with how much I was putting in my mouth for a week. I did. Next appointment was in the clear. Don't avoid weight gain, don't be scared of weight gain, just be conscious of it for health purposes—for you and your baby.

3 Fixes for Getting Fit with a Bump in Tow
From Sia Cooper, mom, National Academy of Sports Medicine (NASM) certified personal trainer, and founder of DiaryOfAFitMommy.com

I started following Sia on Instagram as a fluke not too long before writing this book—and then I suddenly discovered a scathing article about how so many online haters ripped her apart for exercising (and looking great) during pregnancy and after birth. Sia's backstory inspired me, and I'm so thankful she agreed to share some of her favorite quick fixes for getting fit with a baby bump.

1. **Don't skip the weights!** Weight lifting during pregnancy helps a new mom maintain her muscle memory, which will

help her bounce back quickly after pregnancy. Start light and slowly work your way up to a weight that feels slightly challenging but comfortable.

2. **Cardio is your BFF.** Cardio decreases excess weight gain and aids in fat burn during pregnancy (not the fat you need to make the baby, but the extra, unnecessary fat). It's also been proven to strengthen baby's heart as well as yours.

3. **Stretch the pains away.** Stretching during pregnancy can eliminate those back, sciatic, and round ligament pains that many women deal with. Stretching also helps manage the stress and anxieties of labor while keeping joints and muscles strong for delivery. Another bonus? Stretching keeps the spine aligned and increases freedom of movement.

So what are you supposed to do if you're at the very end of your pregnancy and have already gained 50 pounds or more before you started reading this book? *Don't fret. Don't freak out. Don't curse my name or trash this book.* Get rid of any worry, guilt, and negative thoughts from your mind—right now. This particular philosophy is a mere section of this book and is not going to make or break you when it comes to being a FAB mom. Part of bouncing back, in motherhood and beyond, is accepting and owning your current situation for what it is and making a commitment to swiftly change something *if* you sincerely want to change it. Talk to your doctor and make a plan to start doing what is in your control now and what is healthy for your particular situation. Enjoy the rest of your pregnancy, be thankful for this most incredible gift, and start your bathroom butt-squats as soon as your doctor gives you the all-clear after birth.

Connecting with your body at any stage is a powerful tool to make you physically, emotionally, and mentally stronger. Your body may not be the *exact* same after becoming a mom (mine isn't!), but I'm personally suggesting to make an effort to bounce it back as assertively as you can within the first three to four months. Why? Well, after three to four months postbirth, your intention might wear off . . . just like it does every February if you don't initiate losing the extra pounds from those frosted sugar cookies during the holidays as soon as January hits. Looking in the mirror and seeing someone who resembles your prebaby body (no matter what size your prebaby body was) does affect your self regard postbaby, how you treat others, and how you parent your child. Set yourself up to feel good about you, because you've got a baby to take care of.

Let's clear your head and set up space in your home to get even better prepared . . .

CHAPTER 3
FOCUSING YOUR HEAD &
FIGURING OUT YOUR SPACE

B y default, pregnancy can confuse even the most focused of female brains. You're tired, you're uncomfortable, you're nervous about the unavoidable unexpected and what little control you might have once your baby is born. So, do something about it and control what you *can,* while you can . . . and consider keeping your mouth shut like I did.

The Perks of Secrecy . . .

As I said at the beginning of this story, I was not ready for my first baby. (Hell, I wasn't even ready for the second baby when she made her presence known just nine months after the first one was born.) Per my goal to keep working on television and landing auditions with hopes of booking future work, I kept my mouth shut when it came to sharing my pregnancy with people. The only folks who knew I was with child, both times, up until my belly completely popped around five and a half months, were my very closest family and friends . . . and I unreasonably swore them secrecy for fear word would leak to folks I worked with.

I kept my pregnancy under wraps and under many, many layers of billowing clothing in an effort to appear "not pregnant to the naked eye." Looking back, I now think how sad it was to keep such celebratory times in my life so confidential. But, in retrospect, this choice also made my pregnancy feel shorter—which then seemed to make my bounceback easier. Even though I was physically pregnant, my mind was determined to consider myself unpregnant. (Stick with me here . . .) Many women say that, since we're pregnant for nine months, it usually takes nine months to feel seminormal again. Well, in my delusions, I was only pregnant for about four months, so at four months postbaby, I found myself feeling pretty good. Make sense? Mind games can be twisted, but they sometimes work.

Call it abnormal or absolutely brilliant, but I credit bump-denial as the one thing that prevented me from vomiting all over a television news anchor desk in New York City back in 2011. Just as I began working for CNN as an entertainment reporter in May 2011 (as part of a long auditioning process to be considered as the replacement cohost for cable news network HLN's *Showbiz Tonight*, now off the air), I found out I was expecting another baby. *Keep your mouth shut. Land this job first. As far as anyone knows, you're not pregnant.*

I repeated that mantra in my head as I sat next to host A. J. Hammer with scripts on the glass desk front of me, reading a teleprompter and describing the latest shenanigans of headline maker back then, actor Charlie Sheen. My stomach was upside down, but my face was smiling like a cat who swallowed a canary (who was also ready to upchuck out of my mouth and shout "Surprise, she's pregnant!" at any moment, on air). *Keep carrying on. You're not pregnant.* Denial saved my butt for two days during the most intense career snapshots of my life. It was the second time I'd hid my pregnancy in the name of keeping my priorities sharp, and the second time I'd opt for not finding out the sex of my baby on account of staying level-headed for practical purposes.

Wait, say what? Now you might be thinking, "This chick is insane . . . who doesn't want to know whether they're having a boy or a girl?" You're not wrong, and most of the civilized world agrees with you. However, I will argue that choosing to have control over what I'm going to call the "genderlessness" of your baby can be a most valuable exercise for developing your ability to prioritize what's important and what's not—so that you're a total pro about prioritizing after baby comes. *If you already know the sex of your baby and have already told the whole world online and off, read this section for pure entertainment and scoff at how ridiculous I probably sound to you. I also give you permission to roll your eyes and make snarky comments at the pages, just for kicks.* Now back to the perks of gender secrecy . . .

Not finding out the sex of your baby is an exercise in learning how to take control for when after baby comes. I became notorious for not wanting to know my baby's gender. It annoyed some (my sister), it confused many (my mother-in-law), and made others applaud my old-fashioned efforts (my own old-school mom). My husband and I didn't know if we were having a boy or a girl for each of my pregnancies. Personally, I loved not knowing who was living in my belly. In a warped way, it made me feel like I was in control of my body, my baby, and my personal choices for every-thing pertaining to new parenthood.

Why did I jump for gender surprise? The selfish truth was that I really, really, really wanted to have daughters. Given my vola-tile reaction upon finding out I was pregnant for the first time, I decided I didn't need to know any extra information (like the sex of the baby) for fear it would ignite my emotions in another irrational tangent. (For the record, I have two girls, but you probably already know that. My wicked plan worked.) So, I relinquished control over finding out the sex and discovered how much solace it actually gave me in return.

For starters, registering for a genderless baby was a cinch. There were no big decisions to be made about colors, designs, and on and on—whites, creams, light yellows, and pastel greens were my palettes for any and all baby gear, products, and purchases. All items matched in a very chic way—swaddle blankets, play mats, chairs, towels, and onesies. Boring, you say? (Remember when I mentioned that some of my tricks had costs in the beginning of this book? Maybe you count this nonfun practicality as a cost you can't deal with—fair enough.) While many of my friends got bogged down with the back-and-forths of deciding which color schemes and designs to coordinate for gear and nursery, I was making quick choices left and right and getting on with my life. Doing it this way also guaranteed that most everything I was collecting for Baby #1 would be suitable for potential future babies, even if those future babies turned out to be the opposite sex of my first born. It turned out to be the smarty-pants, money-saving thing to do in the long run . . . for me.

This genderless baby business also grounded everyone else's perspective when it came to gifts I received. Instead of finding myself piled with twenty-five hot-pink tutus *(It's a girl! We couldn't resist!)* or nineteen red-and-blue-train piggy banks *(It's a boy! We couldn't resist!)*, I ended up receiving items I'd *actually need and use* for the day-to-day caring of my baby. When folks don't know the gender, you suddenly get usable items like diapers, bottles, and onesies. Carrying a plain old "baby" pretty much cornered my friends and family into purchasing useful items, which made me feel more prepared, organized, stress-free, and absolutely ready for baby's arrival during my third trimester. I had everything I needed . . . done.

Not knowing my baby's gender nudged me to let go of presuppositions and fears and simply live in the moment, undistracted. Back then, I knew myself well enough to realize that, if I found out the sex of my baby, I'd quickly project all sorts of expectations on my tiny person before they were even born. I didn't want to think about a pink room, a blue room, dance lessons, or baseball practice. I was pregnant with a *baby*—that was all I truly needed to know. Pregnancy is pregnancy. The parenting direction and choices would come later, after the baby was born. Lifestyle experts now identify this most sought-after life skill of living in the moment as "mindfulness." As experts will also attest, mindfulness is a major key to happiness, gratitude, and the ability to successfully cope with life's challenges.

On another note, carrying a genderless baby also got me through the fear of delivery. I was petrified of giving birth. *Petrified.* The suspense and anticipation of a final reveal, whether a delicious boy or sweet girl was living in my belly all those months, proved to be my saving grace and quelled all those immature fears about what really happens in the delivery room on D-Day. Not finding out the sex of my baby focused my head in a most unexpected way, which also spawned a most practical philosophy about what kind of stuff a baby truly needs . . .

Bye-Bye, Baby Gear!

Sorry, baby stores and brands, I do love your modern creativity and offerings, but it is time to bust open the wild truth to expecting and new moms everywhere: you don't really need everything everyone tells you you'll need. It's not that I'm not a fan of baby gear *(I am! Have you seen the stroller that folds by itself and fits under the seat of an airplane?!?! And now, there's a car seat that installs itself with an app that assures you you've done it all right! Amazing!)*, it's just that I've promised you no-nonsense advice, so that's what I'm going to shamelessly deliver.

When you register, whether you know the sex of the baby or not, you must keep these words close, remember them, and maybe even read them aloud as you walk down the aisles:

- ☺ *A baby is a baby. Billions of babies have been born in the world, over thousands of years, and have survived and thrived without half of this crap I'm looking at now.*
- ☺ *I'm not the first woman to ever have a baby.*
- ☺ *A baby needs food, diapers, and a safe place to sleep. (And of course love.)*

Wow. Way to suck all the excitement out of shopping and gawking at the most innovative gear available today. What's the point of my big buzzkill attitude? To keep your perspective rational so you don't 1) overspend your hard-earned cash on a $1,000 stroller that you don't need, 2) clutter your brain and cause yourself stress with trivial dilemmas and decisions involving which kind of changing pad cover truly is "the best," and 3) waste limited time and energy during pregnancy running back and forth to the baby store and/ or selecting, deselecting, and rearranging your online registry over and over because "you're just not sure you picked the right stuff."

Here are the products a baby needs, in order of importance:

- ☺ *A Car Seat*

  Tested and approved to meet US safety standards—you can't take baby home from the hospital without one! Might I suggest opting for a color that matches the interior of your car; not only will it make your decision making easy and come in handy for potential future babies (there's that genderless philosophy again), it will also make you feel less inundated with baby designs on everything you will soon own (because you will have plenty of animals and colors taking over your life later). FAB tip: The most expensive car seat isn't necessarily the best. Do your research, check with the Consumer Product Safety Commission (CPSC), make a choice, and move on with your life.

- ☺ *Lots of Diapers*

  So you know, newborns can use about ten diapers a day. The second you put one on, you may very well be changing it about five minutes later. It is not poor form to register for diapers, because you will use them. Ask your doctor how your baby is measuring toward the end of your pregnancy (how many pounds he/she might guess the baby will be when born) and then purchase and/or register for diapers from there. Ten diapers a day adds up to three hundred diapers for the first month. Best to get a few boxes of a few sizes. FAB tip: Do not be lured into the cloth diaper trap. Yes, it may be better for the environment, but if you're interested in helping the environment, I personally suggest finding another way to do it. Cloth diapering will suck up time and energy you don't have to spare after the baby is born. Best way to change a diaper is to throw it away and never deal with it again.

☺ Swaddling Blankets

Whether you opt for blankets or swaddling zip-up "sacks," make sure you've got four to six of these in your possession by the time baby arrives. Prior to becoming a mom, I had no idea about the whole "fourth trimester, swaddle-your-baby-calm" thing. But man, is it *real*. If you don't know who pediatrician Dr. Harvey Karp is (author of the famous *The Happiest Baby on the Block* books and DVDs), look him up and get your swaddling technique ready. FAB tip: Some new moms will tell you that their babies don't like the swaddle, but it's because they're (most likely) not implementing Dr. Karp's full program of "The 5 S's" correctly. Look him up and do what he says. Trust me. (No, Dr. Karp has not put me up to this . . .)

☺ Onesies

You can collect all the adorable ruffles and jeans and trendy outfits with hats your little heart desires, but your newborn will most likely live in onesies the first few months. If baby is born during a cold climate, plan on registering for eight to ten long-sleeved and/or footed onesies and five to six short-sleeved ones. If baby is born during a hot climate, get eight to ten short-sleeved onesies and call it day. (Know that these numbers are created with the assumption that you'll be doing laundry about every other day, which you will with a baby.) FAB tip: plan for the future on your registry by also requesting the next larger sizes. I requested Newborn, 3–6 months, 6–9 months, and even a few 12-month sizes in onesies, according to what age my babies would be in which seasons.

☺ A Stroller

Finding a stroller is similar to finding a car seat. You want one that's safe, practical, can fit into your car, and won't break the bank. Sure, today's stroller designs offer some of the most inspiring tech-savvy features that include self-folding, keeping track of how many miles you've walked (hello fitness buffs!), and all-terrain wheels that will let you hike the most treacherous hills with baby right in front of you. I urge you: be realistic about what you *actually* need and what you can *afford*. FAB tip: Instead of purchasing a "real" stroller, I opted for getting only a stroller frame (that you attach the entire car seat to) and then later got a $120 sturdy-but-basic umbrella stroller for when my daughter started riding around in a sit-up position (around seven months). What's that? You've got lots of money and are absolutely cool with dropping $1,000 on a stroller? Then go for it! Just make your decision fast . . .

☼ A Bassinet

I'm a big believer in keeping a newborn in the parents' room for overnight sleep the first few months, but in a bassinet as opposed to a cosleeper (more on the whys of that later—warning, it's one of those "tough call/costs" I mentioned earlier). FAB tip: Get a bassinet that rolls around on wheels from room to room easily; it'll come in handy when you want to make yourself coffee and watch your baby sleep at the same time.

☼ A Crib

Technically, your baby won't need this until after the first few months, as she will fit in the bassinet for the first two to three months (or, three and a half to four months if you're really lucky) so you technically have a bit of time before you really need a crib set up. However, find your crib (a safe, nonrecalled, and current design approved by CPSC) and set it up anyway to finish the job ahead of time. You'll thank yourself later. FAB tip: Forget the fancy bedding and extra pillows for baby's bedding; you're going to have to remove them anyway for safety. A mattress cover, a fitted sheet, and some safety-approved bumpers are all you need. (Yes, mine were off-white, for my gender-less babies.)

☼ A First Aid Kit

This kit should include a snot-sucker of your choice, baby thermometer, antibacterial ointments, nail scissors, and more random goods. Many of them are prepackaged and ready for purchase at baby stores everywhere.

⊕ *Bottles*

Get large and small sizes. (I got four of each size.) We'll cover more about this topic later (this tip pertains to perhaps the most controversial choice that benefitted me and bounced me back quickly beyond what I ever imagined).

That's it. That's the list of what a newborn *needs*. Obviously, you're going to register and shop for more stuff than this. The only point of this bitchy list was to sharpen your awareness of a *need* versus a *want. Yes! I registered for the big fluffy white lamb floor mat that made me happy all over! Damn right I asked for that video baby monitor! Did I get the wipe-warmer? NO! Babies all over the world have survived without wipe-warmers and mine will, too! Clunky bottle sterilizers aren't necessary—nor do they legitimately sterilize as they're advertised for you to believe—so I opted out of getting that space-sucking contraption, too!* You get my point.

Learn to shop for gear as what you will need versus what the salesperson is trying to sell you. The last thing any expecting mom should have to deal with is a feeling of being overwhelmed by "We need soooooo muuuuuuuuch stuuuuuuuuuuuuff and I can't think straight!" Use your good sense and practical judgment. Will you be a busy working mom who will most likely not have extra time to make your own baby food? Then don't bother registering for a baby food maker. Do you honestly see yourself jogging with baby in that most techy and trendsetting jogging stroller when you don't even jog outdoors now and never did? C'mon. Know yourself (because I know you do). Save yourself time, money, and fretting about things that you're never going to use anyway. Because all that stuff will just make you angry about not having enough space to store it.

3 Fixes for Finding the Right Baby Gear

From Ali Landry, mom, actress, television host

True story: The first crowd I ever spilled the beans to that I was secretly expecting my first baby was at Ali Landry's house, at a beauty party. I was there as a random attendee (thanks to a publicist I was working with at the time). She had no idea who the heck I was when I showed up, but Ali was gracious, welcoming, and soon after became a powerhouse "mompreneur" as cofounder of the FavoredBy.com app and the annual Celebrity Red Carpet Safety Event in Los Angeles—with both resources educating new parents about baby gear and child travel safety. Here are Ali's tips for finding baby gear . . .

1. **Ask around.** Talk to other like-minded moms, with the same lifestyle as you, to see what they like (and what they don't like). Be honest about what you'll really use and what you won't.

2. **Do your research!** Baby products change year to year, and brands are always offering great products to make our lives easier as moms.

3. **Slow down.** Don't worry about getting everything right away. Babies need very few things in the beginning; take your time getting to know your baby and recognizing your new lifestyle. See what products you actually *need* before spending lots of money on things you don't really need.

Now that you know what a real drag I am about shopping for baby, I'll redeem myself. Here's what *you* need as a new mother (a.k.a., the super fun part). Some details describing the reasons for why these things help with a bounceback are described later, throughout the following chapters—I'll just name them and give you a heads-up now. Add the following items to your registry or buy them outright so you're stocked and ready postbirth:

- *A large diaper bag that doesn't look like a diaper bag (so you still feel chic)*
- *Postpartum tummy wrap and/or compression shape-wear*
- *Dry shampoo & tinted root spray*
- *Natural oils/fragrance (because you will most likely not shower every day)*
- *Light-blocking sleep mask (for midday snoozes while baby sleeps)*
- *New sneakers*
- *Cleansing facial wipes (so you don't feel so bad about not washing your face)*
- *Bronzer for body/face*
- *Full-bottomed & high-waisted panties*
- *Thick maxi-pads (I'll let your doc or closest friends explain this one)*
- *3M micropore paper tape (this comes in handy if you have a C-section)*

Don't feel selfish requesting or getting hold of these products. The purpose of a registry is to help the new mother collect goods that will help her care for her baby, and each of these items offers physical comfort and emotional support for the new mom that contribute to caring for the new baby! Side Note: May I also suggest packing your bag for the hospital and cramming it in your closet so that it's ready for action about a month before your due date? I'm guessing you've already looked up and gotten suggestions about what to take? Good. Then I won't bother going there. (Don't forget your phone charger . . . or toothbrush . . . or robe and slippers . . . and lip gloss.)

Now that you've been saved from wasting all sorts of time on things that don't truly matter, let's turn our attention to things that will serve you in the most stress-free way the first few weeks after baby arrives: what the heck you're going to eat for breakfast, lunch, and dinner during your forthcoming newborn lockdown . . .

Food, the Fridge & the Freezer.

Maybe your mom lives next door and has offered to supply your spouse and yourself with breakfast, lunch, and dinner for the first month after baby arrives. Maybe you have a mother-in-law who doesn't have any other grandchildren and will offer the same amenities complete with grocery shopping services. I had neither option. You too? I see.

My mom (who is the original FAB Mom, by the way) lives about two hundred miles away and was able to come stay with us for the first five days after each baby before rightfully needing to head back home to my dad and her responsibilities. My mother-in-law (who lives nearby and graciously makes Sunday night dinner for my husband's brothers and all our families) worked full-time and had legitimate commitments like most folks do the rest of the week. I didn't have a housekeeper or nanny grocery shopping for me. Although my husband now stops at the market on occasion, I don't remember him making regular trips to the grocery store early on in our newlywed adventures. Whether or not either of us ate anything for breakfast, lunch, or dinner was up to me, the new mom trying to figure out how to take care of a baby. Talk about a need to bounce back.

Lucky for me, my mom suggested I "get prepared" before delivery and instructed me to start stockpiling food in our then-apartment during my third trimester. Like a stellar daughter, I listened and started making casseroles. About a month before my due date, I tackled my favorite enchilada making: dipping, rolling, and piling into a pan all that I could jam into the freezer so we were ready for a hot, home-cooked meal after baby—until I thought I was going into labor halfway through my rolling with sticky red sauce smeared all over my white tile countertops.

I remember the squeeze I felt in my insides and around my back. *Oh no no no no. Were these real contractions? I'm going into labor as I'm preparing for life after baby? Does this baby not like enchiladas? Crap.* The thought of going into labor with my husband still at work spooked me a bit, but I was more worked up about the thought of having to dash to the hospital without having time to clean up all the shredded cheese and red sauce smeared all over the place. *Do I have time to rinse the dirty pans? Or would I just leave them on the stove to crust and mold and run out the door?* I pictured us returning home days later with our newborn and wastefully having to throw away my brand new cookware because of the filthy condition I'd left them in. I stupidly started crying. (Hormones.) Turns out those contractions were the "minipractice ones" that ob-gyns tell you about—they came and went, and I continued to roll tortillas. I baked and froze my casserole. I cleaned my kitchen. The next day, I think I made lasagna.

I've always loved cooking, which is why I made and froze a few homemade things as a stress reliever during my last month of pregnancy, but my red sauce experience gave me stress I didn't need.

Homemade casseroles can be useful after baby, but having real food supplies are useful, too. Lesson learned. I changed my game plan to get our future food situation under control. Yes, we could've ordered food from local spots and asked friends to bring meals over for the first few weeks postbaby, but being burdened with the coordinating (that would inevitably fall on me) seemed like more trouble than the alternative. So, I decided to take charge and load up. What did I do first? I hunted and gathered anything I could keep in the cupboards.

It took a few trips to the grocery store with a thirty-seven weeks belly, but I bought enough nonperishables to last us about a month. Never in my life did I have more pasta (traditional and whole wheat), rice (white and brown), quinoa (traditional and red), canned beans (black, kidney, garbanzo, great white, barbeque with maple sauce), crackers of all varieties (love my Wheat Thins), dry cereals, oatmeal, granola, canned fruits and vegetables in their own juices (tomatoes, corn, pears, peaches, pineapples are about all I can stand canned). We could've survived the apocalypse.

I didn't stop there. Let's not forget that "nonperishables" also include paper towels, napkins, toilet paper, dishwashing detergent, laundry soap, shampoo, cleaning agents, tissues, over-the-counter medications, basic makeup I happen to wear every day . . . you're going to need and want all that stuff accessible with a new baby in the house. Basically, think of everything you use to keep your home, your spouse, and yourself clean and comfortable and buy it before you hit thirty-six weeks pregnant. Do you have enough deodorant? Are you running low on toothpaste? Stock up so you don't have anything home-related to stress about for the first month of baby's life. Now that most of us take great advantage of shopping online, we don't have any excuses for not being prepared for the kind of home lockdown a baby can bring.

With all my new toilet paper and spaghetti put away, I then started stocking my freezer with breads, meats, and frozen fruits and vegetables. Frozen produce retains similar (if not very close to the same) fiber, mineral, antioxidant, and carbohydrate content as fresh produce. I had enough frozen peas, green beans, corn, raspberries, peaches, cherries, blueberries, and strawberries stashed to soothe enough bruises and black eyes for an entire football team. (That's not a joke.)

Frozen produce is already cleaned, chopped, ready for fast cooking (pop it in the microwave or dump in in a skillet!) and deliciously filling if you throw it in a blender with yogurt and juice or milk and whip up a smoothie. FAB tip: If you're into it, almond milk can be purchased at almost any grocery store—at room temperature, in a carton—and lasts for about six months (keep in mind that once you open it, you must refrigerate and drink it within seven to ten days, but the storage life before opening it is impressive).

Isn't this too dramatic—stocking up all this food? Bulking up on the items you're able to healthfully store ahead of time—before you're distracted by a new baby's needs—makes you feel calm, organized, and in control with time to spare before baby comes. And, unless you've already found out firsthand, this kind of semi-obsessive behavior to organize and control just before birth is called "nesting." It's a real, evolutionary thing that we can't help but do late in pregnancy—so why not make the most of it with food prep!

Why can't you just clean out drawers (for nesting) and then just order takeout after baby comes? Because eating nonrestaurant food is healthier and better for your body's bounceback. What's that? You have a spouse who is a whiz in the kitchen and does all the shopping to being with? Well now I'm just envious that you don't have to worry about any of this. Send that man on a hunt-and-gathering quest to store food for the winter! (Way to go, woman!)

But, if you're like me, you might have a gem of a guy who doesn't find joy in hitting the market.

The other perk of stepping up and stockpiling ahead of time is that it leaves very few perishable items for your other half to easily pick up when duty calls. "Can you grab a gallon of milk, a head of lettuce, and a few yogurts before you come home, babe?" Compare that to "We have nothing to eat in this house! Can you go to the store and load up everything. . . . I'm just hungry and tired and unclean and don't want to load the baby up to do it." Now, I don't know about your spouse, but if you send my darling husband to the grocery store with an expectation of getting some kind of complete grocery sampling, you'll end up with chipotle corn nuts, dried seaweed, blue raspberry licorice, and a pint of milk. And then, everyone's cranky: you're cranky because you're hungry, and your spouse is cranky because of how snippy you got when you saw what he brought home. Not ideal. (More about enlisting a reluctant spouse to help with the baby duties later . . .)

FAB tip! On scoring more food . . .

Preparing for meals is a must in the last weeks of pregnancy, but don't forget about asking for food from your friends. That's right, see if you can convince your BFF to organize and get a meal train going to inspire friends and family to bring you a meal for the first month postbirth. Get six friends or family members—those who come to your baby shower, people you work with, your neighbors, etc.—and you've got at least one meal accounted for each week. Beg your friend to pull this together, swear her to secrecy, and then pretend you have nothing to do with it if anyone asks you. . . .

As for that shopping list to fill in the blanks between your pasta and rice stockpile? Here are some tested, good-mood foods to keep in mind for your list of needed perishables after baby. Text this quick list, along with "get milk too," to your spouse to pick up:

- 🍼 *Eggs:* High-quality protein, rich in amino acids to promote feelings of well-being
- 🍼 *Asparagus:* Rich in fiber with diuretic properties, can improve digestion and metabolism
- 🍼 *Wild Salmon, Mackerel, Herring:* Contain omega-3 fatty acids and have been shown to stabilize moods and relieve anxiety
- 🍼 *Watermelon & Natural Coconut Water:* Full of natural electrolytes and good for hydration and reducing irritability
- 🍼 *Bananas:* Loaded with potassium for helping with concentration and alertness
- 🍼 *Natural (live) Yogurt:* Packed with probiotics and believed to lower stress hormones in the blood
- 🍼 *Turkey:* Contains amino acid tryptophan and promotes serotonin production (a happy hormone)

Compare the benefits of this market list with blue raspberry licorice. (Not that there's not a place for blue raspberry licorice . . .)

3 Fixes for Fabulous Fast Food

From Catherine McCord, mom, author, and founder of Weelicious.com & One Potato food delivery

I met Catherine about four months after my first daughter was born—I was hired to interview her for a digital series about inspiring women who were moms and businesswomen. She was a spitting image of actress Cameron Diaz and wonderfully friendly. Years before, when her older children were babies, Catherine launched her signature Weelicious site and has grown to be the go-to mom for fast and healthy family food recipes and resources. I'm thrilled to share her tips here . . .

1. **Freeze bananas!** In the last two months when you're in nesting mode, peel, slice, and freeze overripe bananas in plastic baggies to go into those delicious and nutritious smoothies you'll be blending and downing to stay hydrated (for breastfeeding and/or general postpartum health). Makes for a fast and healthy breakfast that will keep you full.

2. **Chill the griddled goods.** If you make pancakes or waffles before baby, you can place a few in zipper bags and freeze them for up to four months. These can easily be popped into the toaster or microwave to quickly reheat.

3. **Veggies are cool.** Frozen vegetables are a lifesaver! Never turn up your nose at them, as they're picked at the peak of perfection and frozen to retain their nutrients. Keep as many as you can in your freezer leading into those postpartum months to toss into stir-frys and soups, mix with rice or pasta, or just to eat them on their own for extra nutrition and energy.

Use your freezer, abuse your cupboards in the best way, employ your ability to plan ahead, and your fridge will be full of food to serve you well for the first month or more after baby arrives. A fast bounceback can't happen if everyone's hungry and unprepared. And speaking of cranky, I cooked up a little letter for the fathers to read ahead of the birth. You know, just as a fabulous FYI. Dads, this next part is for you . . .

DEAR DADS:
A FRANK LETTER FOR FATHERS

Dear New Dad,

First of all, congratulations! You're going to be great. Amazing. The best. Now that we've gotten that out of the way, I'm going to respectfully ask that you listen here:

Your wife might temporarily flip out a bit when the baby comes. Don't panic.

What do I mean? I mean that she might get really tired, be in physical pain, feel awkward and uncomfortable in her new role as mom, act more sensitive than usual, become unexpectedly bossy, request certain things that she never requested before, say no to certain things—and then get angry about things she never said no to before. (I certainly did.) Please, just give a free pass the first few months or so and listen to her. Why? A baby brings change—adjustment to change can sometimes spark arguments. Don't be scared of it, just be aware so it doesn't blindside you.*

Here's a personal story for the books (well, for this book anyway): When my first baby was born, I sort of "hated" my husband for about a month. Okay, I didn't *really* hate him, but I felt frustrated and angry because of our different perspectives about postpartum life, new babies, and appropriate involvement from extended family. It made for an interesting first month. Keep in mind, my husband and I were this sappy, lovey-dovey, always-holding-hands couple who'd just gotten married about a year before becoming parents. I was *in love* with my husband. My own family used to tease me about how in love I was with him. (I still am in love . . .)

Well, even though my husband and I share the same cultural background (Armenian), I soon found out that his family had very different opinions and practices from my own when it came to new babies' debuts—I'm now finding this is common with many couples. I come from the kind of family that always gave a new mother tons of time and space postdelivery—time and space to return home from the hospital, to organize, to bond privately with her new baby, to calm her wits and adjust herself back to regular life before welcoming guests. Then, in about a week's time, it was all clear to visit the new baby and parents in short and quiet one-hour increments that didn't involve toddlers.

The day I returned home from the hospital, I found myself in a blurry haze of recuperating from heavy induction medication and a fresh and painful C-section incision while welcoming three adults and three young children into our apartment—keep in mind that my mom, my sister, and her husband were already there at the same time, too (because my family lives out of town and they had nowhere else to go). As a first time and semifreaked-out mom who genuinely likes to feel "together" and "prepared" for visiting company of any kind, I was not on board with this large group visitation just after getting home. "Can we just wait a few days? Can they come at a different time?" I kept asking. My husband disagreed and overruled me. "Everyone's excited and this is what my family does . . . they're coming today," he said. Okay then. (Keep in mind that my in-laws had already met the baby at the hospital . . .) Let's just say my husband and I had some arguments the first few days with our new baby.

I love and respect my husband's family, but on that particular day, I was not mentally prepared for noise, excitement, disruption of peace, getting dressed to look halfway decent, and all the things that go with several adults and kids being in my small home at one time. I was on major medication from my C-section and had climbing postpartum high blood pressure that was making my doctor a little nervous. I tried to be cool, as this was family. And, family brings love. *Just chill, Jill.*

I soon started fuming when an impromptu photoshoot—that involved passing my five-day-old newborn around from person to person, child to child—happened without even a request in my direction. I stood by, started to object, and was ignored. (I was so confused.) This was my first baby . . . *our* first baby. And, we've all heard stories about how many first-time moms feel about their first babies—nervous, protective, and majorly territorial. All those things were true for me the first time around. Whatever happened to being kind and respectful to the brand new, semi-freaked-out mother?

My husband's family is wonderful (truly!), and I know they had no idea I was feeling all of these things—they probably would've behaved differently had they known what was going on inside my head. But I stood there behind the couch, watching and feeling like an outsider as my husband snapped picture after picture, repositioned everyone taking turns holding the baby (without asking or including me, by the way), and then snapped away again. I carried those toxic feelings with me for a very, very long time.

Looking back, I now realize that 1) everything was done out of love and excitement for the new baby, 2) that is how my husband's family welcomes a newborn, 3) nothing was technically unsafe, and 4) my anger was ignited and intensified because that was my very first child and I was not yet comfortable with even having a baby, much less watching people pass her around like she was a platter of cookies. No one was right, no one was wrong . . . everyone was right, everyone was wrong. But, in that moment, I hated my husband for not listening to me.

Why did I tell you this? Don't let this happen to you, New Dads. Please, listen to your Baby-Mama's wishes . . . even if you think she's weird and confused and acting like a real witch. Listen to her—pretend to listen to her and nod your head yes if you must. Nothing about having a baby, and what happens the first few weeks after, is rational. Opt to honor what makes the new mother of your child feel comfortable, in control, and happy. If she's not in the mood to see folks one day after getting home, respect that. Explain it to your friends and family and apologize if you must. It just might save you from some major bumps at home those first few weeks.

Think about it. Best of luck . . . and congratulations again!

Sincerely,
Jill

*P.S.: A bit of nerves and baby blues are completely normal for all new moms, thanks to the body and brain's natural hormone readjustment postbirth. However, should you notice your spouse displaying extreme signs of having feelings of hopelessness, deep sadness, and confusion without end or new and obsessive habits that are unlike anything she did before baby in the months following birth, gently suggest opening a discussion with your partner and her doctor about possible postpartum depression and anxiety (yes, it's a real scientific thing). Don't hesitate to ask for help.

PART 3
BREAKING IN
THE BIRTH MONTHS
(Delivery through Month 3)

"What happens with me is that I hear of a great thing and I want to try it. . . . I drank a ton of water, tried acupuncture and flower essences for baby blues. I even did the placenta encapsulation. I literally would've fried it up [the placenta] in a pan if you told me that was the best way to do it . . ."
—Ali Landry, mom, actress & television personality (September 2015)

This is it. It's time. We're having a baby. I think we have to go to the hospital. My water just broke. It's time for our induction appointment. Call the doctor! (Insert glee, panic, elation, dread, tears of joy, tears of fear, and everything else in between here.) No matter how it all begins, you can't slow down The Birth Months once they kick into action. But here's the catch:

it is during this time when you must stop and consciously make some choices. Because how you choose to handle this most fleeting time, beginning from the labor and delivery of baby and into the days and weeks following until baby's three-month birthday, will set a standard for the way you navigate motherhood going forward.

Some women have a deep support system of family and friends close by to help them, some don't. Some women have access to and budget to hire postpartum doulas (whose paid jobs are to help a mother adjust to life with a new baby for a designated amount of time after delivery), and some women don't. Whatever resources you might have or currently be investigating to tap into, there will always be one person you must depend on no matter what help you have from anyone else: you. How to actively learn to depend on yourself during this most confusing time of becoming a new mom? Let's start with your brain . . .

CHAPTER 4

YOUR BIRTH BRAIN

Remember our chat about resilience back in the beginning? Here's where it all slams together and becomes relevant. Your baby's birth is the time to set yourself up to be as stress-free as humanly possible. Let me repeat that: make the choice to be as stress-free as possible—because it *is* a choice. Tap into some mindful breathing techniques or quiet meditation if you have to, but be aware of how much stress you allow into your mind during this time. Face your fears head on, just like the scientists suggest.

Make the Choice to Mom Up.

You have a natural birth plan. You want a C-section. You've requested ahead of time that no one offer you an epidural no matter how you might be tempted to change your mind in the moment. You secretly wish you could be sedated when your baby is born, only for the sake of missing any and all pain. Whatever you're thinking and planning and plotting for your most perfectly ideal birth, throw it out the car window on the way to the hospital. Now is the time to trust the process as it unfolds through the moments, in real time. This includes trusting your doctors, nurses, medical professionals, and/or midwives/doulas, who, frankly, know more about birthing babies than you do. That's not to say you shouldn't listen to your body (you should!), but in this section, Mom-ing Up means letting go and trusting those you've selected to trust for the delivery.

I know, I know. You've read the best material. You've heard the horror stories from your friend's cousin's husband whose sister had a terrifying experience with a bossy substitute ob-gyn during an emergency C-section that she didn't want. You're scared of being pumped with drugs that have been inconclusively questioned and incorrectly correlated with causing autism, developmental delays, and who knows what else because, well, *what if those far-fetched and unproven ideas happen to be true?* As you already know, I come from The Land of Hollywood and Free-Spirited Los Angeles Love, where I know more mothers who encapsulate their own placentas, have home births in bathtubs, and refuse any kind of labor medication at all costs in the name of birthing a pure and natural child. More power to those women (seriously, I mean that) but that ain't my personal style.

If these things aren't your style, either, I'm here to give you exclusive permission to release yourself from any burden of guilt that may hang over you about wanting epidurals or welcoming traditional hospital assistance. Delivering a baby—no matter how it happens—is best accomplished when the mother approaches the process with open confidence, positive faith, and the ability to listen to medical professionals who are more experienced and educated in the field than she. (If you happen to be an ob-gyn yourself, you've got this part aced, baby!) I'm not arguing that highly incompetent medical professionals don't exist (because they do), but the chance that you're going to have an entire delivery team of doctors, nurses, assistants, anesthesiologists, practitioners, and anyone else whom you've enlisted, like a doula or midwife-type, who are all equally incompetent is slim. No matter what you might feel or what fears race through your mind, you must fight to keep a levelheaded mindset throughout your birth. Medical professionals are not out to get you.

Contrary to what some contemporary childbirth connoisseurs may sway you to believe, hospitals and doctors are not interested in risking the health of you or your baby because 1) it's just scary, and 2) they've got legal watchdogs monitoring their every move, ready to take away their medical licenses. One hasty mistake can cost millions of dollars and bring down an entire hospital in one clean swoop thanks to an independent, not-for-profit organization called The Joint Commission that regulates, accredits, and certifies more than 21,000 hospitals and health-care organizations across the United States. Look up this organization—and then search for your hospital to make sure they're accredited (chances are your hospital is; if it's not, consider finding other birthing options). No doctor in his or her right mind—old school, new age, arrogant, or indecisive—wants to mess with The Joint Commission and lose his or her ability to practice.

Educating yourself about the childbirth process, learning what options and rights you have as a woman giving birth, and acting as your own advocate (should something truly feel wrong) is a smart and necessary weapon in this modern age of information, but also keep a rational tab on yourself when it comes to questioning medical insight. *(Ha! Tell my hormones to be rational!)* Recognize the misinformation that can be found on Google and seek value in knowing when it's time to stop putting up a fight because your baby's not being born "like you wanted him to be born." Best way to instigate a bad birthing experience is to pick an argument over something you truly don't know anything about.

But what if my doctor wants to do a C-section when I get there and I don't want a C-section? So what. Big deal. *You mean, you're telling me to abandon my instincts and gut feelings about what's right and wrong for my body?* No, I'm suggesting (okay, fine, telling you) to keep an open mind to trained professionals' insight in the name of delivering a healthy baby. If a C-section presents the option to have a safer and better delivery, then so be it. By all means, ask your doctor all the whys and hows about the risks he or she is trying to avoid and then *listen* to what you're being informed of from a non-threatening, nonconfrontational place. Choose to check your ego at the door . . . and then get over it.

With my first baby, I was adamantly against inducing labor. Four days past my due date, I remember fielding questions from friends and family: "When are you inducing? Are you going to induce? Does your doctor want to do a C-section?" I wanted to tell everyone to shut up and mind their own business. I wasn't inducing, and I certainly wasn't going to do a C-section just for kicks, despite my very real and extreme dread of birthing a baby the way nature intended. My doctor mentioned the possibility of induction at my final appointment, but as much as I adored her and valued her knowledge and experience, I opted to kindly ignore the option. "Let's just wait," I said. "Can we wait?" She agreed to wait for a few days. I was happy.

I've always believed in letting the body do its thing—labor will happen when it's physiologically ready to happen, according to my body and my baby. (Although I was intent on getting an epidural, know that I'm also the woman who resists taking any kind of pain reliever for a headache because I'm convinced my body will reset to being pain-free naturally. Drives my surgeon-husband nuts.) I've always trusted that a healthy human body is a well-oiled machine that takes care of itself, and I was going to stick to my guns unless a real medical risk required me to do otherwise. Or, until my husband strapped me to a Pitocin drip against my will.

I Googled "Ways to Induce Labor" and found every suggestion from have sex to drink castor oil to take a long walk to stimulate your breasts. I even bullied my husband into hauling me to a local restaurant that boasted a legendary labor-inducing salad that a friend of mine told me to try. The place was famous in Los Angeles and had been featured in all sorts of newspapers and magazines—the spices in the salad dressing allegedly had a history of kick-starting contractions. Hundreds of pregnant women traveled over the years from far and near to eat this magical dish and then reportedly went into labor hours later. I decided to try it in the name of not wanting to induce labor.

I was beyond giddy when we got there. My husband laughed and rolled his eyes. I signed the mommy-to-be guestbook, ordered the salad with a wild psychotic smile on my face, and waited for my contractions-on-a-plate to arrive. I dug in. I had a delicious, crunchy bite dripping with the tangy-sweet dressing, looked down to go in for more, and then spotted a tiny surprise squirming between a cucumber and tomato: there was a larva-looking worm thing working its way through my lettuce! I gagged and almost vomited right there. (An innocent mishap—I do *not* hold the restaurant responsible, but I shiver every time I think about it now.)

Maybe the bug hung on through washing the lettuce, maybe it fell from the ceiling while the cook was tossing in the dressing, maybe my unborn child willed it there from the womb because she was not ready to be born yet? We sent my salad back and ordered a pizza. The waitress apologized and gave me some dressing to take home and have later, which I did, but no labor. The freak I am, I took this as a sign from God and The Universe not to tamper with the labor and delivery process. I was soon forced to Mom-Up and let go.

Two days later, my doctor called to playfully ask where our baby was. She started revisiting options about how and when we were going to get my stubborn little nugget out should he or she refuse to appear in the next few days. At one week overdue with absolutely no progress whatsoever, it was looking like my doc was going to prevail victorious in her push for Pitocin before I reached two weeks overdue. Now I was starting to get pissed off.

I whined about wanting to wait until things progressed naturally. I prayed my water would miraculously break. I worried and complained how things were not going my way, how I knew my body best, and how I was beginning my journey as a mother with an opposite philosophy from how I'd lived my life so far. My husband was starting to lose major patience with me. I felt stress . . . lots of stress. Then, just when the topic was super hot and I sensed controlled frustration coming from my ob-gyn, she finally told me about certain risks that can multiply about one to two weeks after a past-due date called postmaturity syndrome, which basically means the placenta stops working effectively. (Yes, I Googled this, too, and also asked my husband about it. Contrary to his ongoing annoyance with the Internet's ever-present promotion of self-diagnosis, he backed up that this risk was in fact valid.) The second I read how some postmaturity studies indicate increased risk of developmental problems in newborns, I decided to let go of my preconceived notions about induction and just trust my doctor.

A few days later, the Pitocin drip found me. My labor progressed quickly, I dilated just as expected, I got that epidural . . . and then everything stalled for about eight hours. I stopped dilating and progressing. We waited and waited. Then, my baby's heartbeat started to show distress every time I moved. Nurses flipped me on my side. They flipped me on my other side. They strapped an oxygen mask on my face to make sure baby was getting enough air. No more dilation, no more progression, no more simple answers. Hour ten rolled around. My doctor kept monitoring me, turning me over and around and doing all those medical-things to figure out the best solution. I wasn't in pain, and I didn't feel like anything was terribly wrong (minus the oxygen mask and the constant beeping from the machine I was hooked up to, tracking inconsistencies in baby's heartbeat).

My doctor then sat on my bed and looked at me with the most somber expression I'd ever seen from her. My heart stopped in fear. *Oh no. What now. What's happened?* "Jill, how do you feel about a C-section? I think it's the smartest way to go." Without hesitation, I responded, "Yes. Do it. Get the baby out." That was easy. "Do it," my husband said (but operations are no big deal to him).

Mom-Up. Let Go. It's Okay.

Unexpectedly having a C-section seemed a hell of a lot better than traumatically struggling to birth a baby with an unstable heartbeat thanks to an umbilical cord wrapped around her neck. *Get the baby out safely. Your doctor is trained to do this.* I quickly got over my ignorant opinions about what was right and wrong during childbirth. I was happy to take a C-section scar and forfeit the body's natural process if it meant giving my baby a low-risk birth. My daughter was delivered safely and healthy and developed perfectly normally despite not moving through the birth canal.

As for my second daughter's birth story? Well, she sent me into contractions about twelve hours before my scheduled C-section. We rushed to the hospital, found out I was significantly dilated, and the doctors did a "rush" C-section right then and there. Talk about letting it all go . . .

---

3 Fixes for Comfort & Healing After a C-section.

From Dr. Andre Panossian, plastic & reconstructive surgeon (this smart and sweet guy also happens to be my husband)

I first met Andre at a huge dinner dance and was impressed by his medical accomplishments, but was more fascinated that he consulted for ABC's long-running hit show *Grey's Anatomy* (details about this coming soon, keep reading). After taking care of my C-section stitch in the following way after both babies, I'll shamelessly tell you that my scar is barely visible. Here are a few tips for how we helped pulled that off . . . but be sure to check with your own doctor for details and extra help!

1. **Tape it**. Gently cover scar with 3M micropore paper tape, all the way across the scar (end to end, horizontally) after stitches are out (approximately two to three weeks

---

postsurgery). Lightly pat the tape on and keep it clean with mild soap and water (yes, you can shower with it). When it starts peeling on the ends from natural wear, remove the entire piece with baby oil and secure a new piece of tape on top of scar again. Repeat for two months, as tape will encourage scar to heal flat. (This is a classic plastic surgeon's trick that most general surgeons don't do. Ask your doctor about it postsurgery.)

2. **Cover yourself.** Wear a postpartum tummy wrap (as described in the following sections); the corset-like design helps with postsurgery support for the core. Consider getting high-waisted, postpartum undergarments that offer silicone strips that lay on top of the front of the belly. The silicone will comfort the stitches and scar.

3. **Moisturize.** Use scar cream as directed (although, the 3M micropore paper tape works much better, in my opinion). There are many available over the counter, but if you've got the means, there are also prescription-level options available. Ask your ob-gyn.

Did I cry and feel like a failure for not doing things as I'd initially planned? Did I feel guilty or cheated by the childbirth gods for having a C-section? Nope. Was I in physical pain afterward? Of course, but you can't escape that no matter which way a baby busts into the world. Part of staying focused and fabulous after having a baby is accepting that you must sometimes put your big girl panties on, let any change in plans roll off your back, and continue on to life's next big thing, whether or not it bothers you. Mental strength always weakens physical pain (easier said than done, I know). Just because something doesn't go the way you planned doesn't mean it's a failed endeavor. Which leads me to say . . .

F-Off to the F-Word!

Our naughty F-word here is (drumroll): Fail. Drop any other F-bombs you want, but this F-word is the dirtiest one you can think or say during your first days and weeks as a new mom. From this point forward, make a promise to yourself that you will not use that most destructive word as you forge ahead into motherhood. However your baby was born, whatever you did or didn't do, Mom-Up with a positive attitude and commit to making decisions free of regret, guilt, or feelings of failure that will haunt your thoughts. As innocently as you might say this F-word to lighten a disappointing or frustrating situation, the word *fail* will kill a bounceback so fast, you won't know what hit you.

When my first daughter was about seven months old, I was one of the cohosts of a fresh little digital series called *Her Say* that was featured on MSN.com during the summer of 2011 with super famous mom blogger, DIY diva, social media powerhouse, businesswoman, and actress Soleil Moon Frye. As a freak-fan of her popular 1980s sitcom *Punky Brewster* when I was a kid, I was elated about sitting next to my childhood idol to talk all things mom and family with millions of viewers watching online every week. Soleil was always cool and collected—she knew who she was and was always so honest and articulate about the topics we'd discuss on camera, whether we were talking about celebrity kids' extravagant tree houses or the pains of labor. But, on one particular day, something she said to our producer during our off-camera, between-scenes chats jarred me and made me think about the real power of words we use.

We were sitting on our stools on set, talking about raising kids and balancing work and home life, and the following words burst out from her mouth: "I just feel like I'm failing all the time . . ." I was confused. *She feels like she's failing? She's like, Supermom! If she's failing, then what hope is there for the rest of us?* At the time, Soleil was a mom of two daughters (who were remarkably polite and sweet the few times they came to set, by the way). She was juggling her explosive site Moonfrye.com, launching her book *Happy Chaos*, developing lifestyle brands and services in the crafty-mom market, and, by all my outsider observations, killing it at work and family life in the best way possible. I admired her tenacity and creativity while raising a young family and accomplishing goals simultaneously. Yet there she was, saying that she felt like she was failing. For all I know, that was the only time in her life she actually said those words, but they affected me so much in that flash.

Her quote that day brought two things to my attention going forward: 1) Every mom feels the same way at one point or another, whether that mom happens to be famous or not, and 2) I soon started noticing more regular, new moms around me using the word *fail* as part of their everyday vernacular. *Mom fail! I feel like a failure for not breastfeeding for the full year. I'm failing at keeping my head on straight. I'm failing at my relationship with my spouse.* Every time I'd hear this offbeat F-bomb, I'd get irritated and offended in the name of supporting capable women everywhere. *Are we all inevitably failing?* Way to bring down our collective self-esteem.

But all moms joke about failing. It's okay to say we fail, it doesn't mean anything. Well, true . . . sort of. Words do start to mean something the more we continue to say them. The more power you give a word, albeit unintentionally, the more power that word has over you, over all of us. Positive words can do great things; negative words can be sneaky about bringing us down, even if we do use them in jest. I happen to be fascinated when it comes to psychology surrounding words, so I asked my friend Katie Hurley, licensed clinical social worker, family psychotherapist, and author of one of my most favorite and helpful books, *The Happy Kid Handbook*, to give me some F-word insight.

Here's what Katie said: "Can the term be used in a humorous way? Yes. Laughter and sarcasm are natural defense mechanisms used to cope with situations that make us feel anxious, guilty, or disappointed. We joke to deflect the feelings and lighten the mood. Venting can be useful, but in small doses. Talking about the lows and commiserating with other moms, either in person or online, normalizes the ups and downs of parenting."

But Katie also recognized how constant negativity can take a toll on our sense of self, even if the word *fail* is tossed around with a sarcastic sneer and giggle. "Moms can get stuck in a negative loop if they only ever see the downsides. This can leave moms feeling overwhelmed and cause their self-esteem to plummet. Constant venting of negative emotion can trigger a cycle of negativity. I don't believe in parenting fails." See? (Told you I liked Katie.) The more we use certain words, the more we believe them to be true.

Growing up, my mom didn't allow my sister and me to say the word *bored* or *boring*. We'd literally get in trouble if either one of us said the B-word. "What did you say?!?" she'd shout from the other room. (It was like we'd said the real B-word or something.) "If you're bored, then find a way to fix it, something to do, to not be bored," she'd matter-of-factly pronounce. So, my sister and I would be forced to find a way to not be bored. Maybe being the educator that my mom is (a teacher), she knew that saying a word repeatedly gives that word power . . . or, she just didn't want to raise brats who couldn't help themselves and solve their own issues. Consider this "no F-word policy" a reincarnation and passing-along-to-you of my mom's most unconventional and motivating problem-solving process back in the day. F-off to negativity. F-off to destructive words. F-off to curbing our own resilience.

Joking that your birth plan was a failure, that you failed to prepare your home or your baby's nursery to the extent you wish you had before your water unexpectedly broke, or even poking fun about how you've "failed" to get dressed in something other than pajamas the first few weeks of becoming a mom promotes a kind of unproductive uncertainty that no new mom should have to deal with. Thinking of yourself as a failure leads to guilt, guilt leads to self-doubt, self-doubt leads to low self-esteem, low self-esteem leads to an inability to function confidently . . . and before you know it, everything's gone to hell in a handbasket, and you can't figure out how to stop your baby from crying.

Not being able to function confidently negatively affects our potential to be good parents. Being a parent is your job now, and you must not ever think you're failing at it. Would you ever stomp around your workplace saying you were failing as an employee? Does a CEO of a corporation go around saying they're failing all their employees and the marketplace around them? Not usually. Remember, creating a believable perception is halfway to creating the truth. Create your truth as a successful new mom with know-how. *No fails happening here.*

Had I started my own motherhood consumed in self-doubt—*I failed by inducing labor! I failed by having a C-section!*—my confidence and capability as a new mom would've been diminished.

I'm not saying to not laugh about all the hysterical circumstances pregnancy and new motherhood can bring (wait until you hear my story about putting frozen cabbage leaves inside my bra and spending full weeks in only my underwear); just be aware of the power of word selections and how they influence actions.

The sooner you recognize the hazard and negative impacts of using that F-word, and make a choice to not use it day in and day out, the better off you'll be. Owning personal triumphs and telling yourself that you're doing a good job for something brand-new to you (i.e., motherhood) are scary, resilience-building things to do, but they're musts (there's that facing-your-fears thing again). Tell the word *fail* to F-off on your way to the hospital, because you've got a list of to-dos ahead of you . . .

Sanity Secrets: Swaddling & Scheduling.

Birthing a baby can be flat-out insane. The first few days and weeks following can and most likely will be a total blur. Amid the rushing adrenaline and most wondrous *OMG who is this precious new person . . . we just love her so much* feelings, your mind might also be pegged with questions. How to launch and support your own sanity from the get-go? Get yourself and your new family on a locked-down, to-do schedule. This thirty-day lockdown, as I call it, is just a frank, no-frills method to get you to focus on your new job at hand—figuring out baby.

How to initiate lockdown? Start by taking full advantage of what your hospital offers you:

- *Request that your baby sleep in the nursery overnight—not in your room.*

"But I just don't want him away from me. . . . He's so precious. . . . I want to savor him right by my side through the night in these glowing first days." I know it's hard, but resist this trap of novel sweetness for the overnight hours if your hospital has a nursery. You need your sleep right now, especially in these first few days immediately after delivery. Regardless of how alert and empowered you feel (coming from someone who felt freakishly invincible and had more energy than expected the day after delivering both my girls), send the baby to the nursery at night and let your body begin its healing process through quality, restorative sleep. The nurses can take care of your pride and joy overnight; they're trained for it. Let them do their job so you can begin to recover. Baby can stay in your room all day, but back to the nursery for bedtime. (NOTE: Some hospitals across the country are eradicating baby nurseries. Check with your local hospital to see if they still have one before your due date.) But what about nursing at night, you ask? Ah. Stay tuned . . . and brace yourself.

☺ *Stay in the hospital for as long as possible—for the longest time your insurance allows and/or you're able (natural births are usually discharged after one to two days, C-sections frequently allow for three to four days).*
Even if the food is crap, even if you're out of clean underwear and are stuck wearing those loose mesh things the hospital gives you to cover your privates, even if you just want to get back to your pretty pillows on your own bed (and all your food stashed ready for you in your freezer), stay as long as you can, for healing's sake. Let the nurses bring you your

meds, help with your child, change that channel on the television from *Maury Povich* to *Real Housewives* (speaking from personal experience here) until hospital regulations kick you out for good. Once you're home, you're on your own.

☺ *Take the drugs they give you, as directed exactly.*
Don't get any shady ideas: I'm not suggesting any kind of medicinal abuse. All I'm reminding you to do is follow doctors' orders. If one of your painkillers is prescribed to be taken every four hours, take that medicine every four hours on the dot to get ahead of the pain and keep it at bay (remember, I had a C-section). No need to try and tough anything out the first week after delivery. Be an A+ patient and ask your nurse to detail any and all instructions for medication when you go home, so that you may check your notes in case you don't remember. The last thing you need inhibiting your ability to care for baby is avoidable physical torment.

☺ *Learn from nurses.*
Watch them handle your newborn like a boss. The biggest motivator I got in the hospital was witnessing how my nurses handled my newborn without fear. Contrary to what I thought, babies will not break! What d'ya know! Nurses are your best resource for teaching you the easiest way to hold, turn over, change clothes, and wipe your baby's butt in a most expedited way. FAB TIP: Ask them to teach you and practice swaddling your baby like a real mother (more on this below).

Once you get home, you might be tired, sore, a bit confused, and sweaty (thanks, readjusting hormones). You might cry. Your baby will most likely cry. Your baby might also scream. You might want to scream. You might actually scream. You might cry again, because you're so damn happy and the joy can't contain itself. If you had a long delivery, you might want to just sleep a lot. Your baby will most likely sleep a lot (most newborns do). Your baby will have his days and nights confused, your schedule will have very little rhyme or reason, and your intention to focus might be topsy-turvy. Most women I know (myself included) craved order and organization during these early days—even if they were never order-and-organization types of gals (myself also included; if you take a look inside my junk drawer at home, you'll understand).

How to set up yourself and your baby for long-term sanity? First, you must designate the first few weeks with baby, the first thirty days, as a locked-down "get to know you" period and nothing else. (Trust me, you're probably going to love it . . . hello, new baby in the house!) No matter how much of a ballbuster you were before birth, your mind and body have gone through a lot and need a buffer of time to recuperate.

Commit yourself to thirty days of "nothing but baby"—don't hope, plan, or bank on going anywhere as a first-time mom besides a required doctor's appointment. Accept this thirty-day blackout period for the sole purpose of saving yourself frustrating thoughts of *Life isn't what it used to be and it's confusing!* Your only purpose the first few weeks is to "learn" your baby, just like a CEO might need to learn about the new company she was hired to lead. Setting low expectations for yourself during those first thirty days (related to getting things done) gives you nowhere to go but up.

My friend and colleague Stephanie Simmons, morning traffic anchor for CBS Los Angeles News, opted for what was close to a two-month lockdown after her baby was born in February 2016 . . . without even washing her hair! "Every day, I'd braid my hair or nestle it up into a bun and wrap my head in a scarf. I maybe washed it once a month . . . maybe. Where was I going and who was I trying to impress anyway?" I almost died laughing when Stephanie told me about this—I thought it was brilliantly honest.

She also told me how she chose to hunker down during maternity leave and "be a mom, only and totally" for the first few months without distraction. She shared how "learning her baby" was what she was focused on during that limited amount of maternity leave time. The unexpected perk about not washing her hair? "Once I returned to work (and finally got back to regular washing and styling), people couldn't believe how fabulous my hair looked! I thank my son."

Second tip for organizing the chaos? Start initiating a feed/play/sleep schedule right around the time your baby turns one month old (this is what I did, anyway). Setting a patterned home routine is serious business, mamas. How in the world to do it? Swaddling your newborn through the fourth trimester (the first three months of your baby's life) is your hot ticket.

If you don't already know about the fourth trimester as detailed in Dr. Harvey Karp's previously mentioned best-selling book *The Happiest Baby on the Block*, here's the gist: the first three months after baby is born is essentially an adjustment period for living outside the womb. Prior to delivery, your baby is all squished up, tightly cuddled by your insides, and is used to hearing the loud rushing sound of your body's workings for nine months—blood traveling through your body, the noisy swishing of organs doing their jobs. (All of which, according to Dr. Karp, are louder than a vacuum cleaner!) Being born into the outside world suddenly throws your child into a sudden "Where the hell am I?" response.

As a first-time, pregnant woman who was petrified of how a constantly screaming baby might jack up my mind, I read Dr. Karp's book cover to cover and soaked up all the scientific research, historical reasoning, and step-by-step guides for Dr. Karp's Five S's swaddling technique. Get the book or look him up online, follow his directions exactly as he outlines them, and feel immediately more focused as a new mom—your baby will be content, and you will be in control. A mom's first job is to make our children feel secure, physically and emotionally. And, you guessed it, making babies feel secure encourages them to feel calm (e.g., less screaming bloody murder), which then allows a mom to think more clearly and feel more focused. You see how this works?

Swaddling unequivocally calmed both my babies, even though my girls' temperaments were on opposite ends of the spectrum. From Day One through Month Three, I swaddled like it was my job—well, it was. Arms locked in, tighter than tight. The more snugly wrapped and held sideways (with baby's tummy fully up against my own chest), the swifter the swinging and the louder the shushing, the quicker baby will calm and the calmer your sanity will be. Swaddling worked so well that I started questioning the smarts and judging anyone who claimed it to be futile. With both my girls, people told me how lucky I was to get easy babies. I wasn't lucky; I just followed credible, proven directions from a visionary medical professional and stuck with them. Swaddling correctly and constantly creates a most probable chance for getting an "easy" baby.

"Swaddling didn't work on my baby," some new mothers might tell you. Yes, it's true, all babies are born differently. (Duh.) But after utilizing all of Dr. Karp's practices through my very opposite back-to-back babies, the chances his method will fail you completely is extremely slim. (In other words, those moms probably weren't following his instructions as precisely as directed. And no, I don't work for Dr. Karp in any way. I'm just a superfan because his method is easy and effective.)

Are some babies born with medical conditions, acid reflux, or other ailments that make calming them more challenging? Yes. Some babies *are* more difficult to handle than others (hello, my own second-born child), and that's when our skills of resilience are challenged and either rewarded or defeated. Most doctors and doulas will tell you that babies generally respond favorably to confidence of any kind, and confidence often comes from Mom-ing Up and following directions relentlessly, without using that F-word.

Coupled with swaddling, setting a schedule for baby is imperative for sanity as a mother. Beginning around the one-month birthday, start putting major effort into curating your baby's predictability by teaching him a rotating daily pattern of when it's time to eat, when it's time to sleep, and when it's time to be awake. The most common complaint most new moms have is, "I can't plan anything because my baby is so unpredictable!" Don't let this be you. The reality of setting a schedule is absolutely possible, worthwhile, and will make your home life with a newborn manageable. However, it's up to *you* to stay consistent and get it done.

Twice in two years, people again accused of me of being "lucky" about how my daughters' daily habits did not throw me for a loop. Just like the swaddling thing, it wasn't luck; my daughters' mostly predictable behavior rested purely on me following directions and implementing them vigilantly. By the time each of them reached their one-month birthdays, I started "training" their days into repeating patterns and got all of us organized by maintaining feed/play/sleep cycles daily. I was motivated to get organized thanks to some unsolicited and fabulous advice from Emmy-winning television actress Ellen Pompeo, who plays Meredith Grey on ABC's long-running, hit show *Grey's Anatomy*. (Told you I have a thing for listening to doctors.)

Long before babies were a blip on my mind, my husband served as a medical consultant for *Grey's Anatomy*. It was an on-and-off gig, and occasionally he'd be called to set to observe, take notes, and offer notes (e.g., "That kind of blood-spraying would never happen in a real-life surgery . . ."). When I was in my eighth month of first-time pregnancy, Andre got called to the show for a random set visit. At the time, Ellen had just had her first baby, so he told her how we were expecting our first in the next month. According to my husband, she was amazingly congratulatory and insistent that I reach out to her for any insight I might be seeking about pregnancy or a new baby. She gave him her email address and then suggested I consider getting my hands on *The Contented Little Baby* book, which had been gifted to me, but I hadn't read yet.

Despite the fact that I'd never met her, I sent Ellen an email introducing myself and thanking her for suggesting I take a peek at that book. She immediately responded with how effective the book's theme of putting baby on a strict schedule was, and how combining the commitment to create a feed/play/sleep schedule with my own instincts on a day-to-day basis (to do what would be best for my child in the moment) was most helpful and calming. Being the Hollywood-loving, direction-following gal that I was, I listened and did what she said. Baby #1 was on a schedule by four weeks old, and Baby #2 was on a schedule somewhere after her first-month birthday (maybe even closer to her second-month birthday, because that's just what happens most of the time with a second kid).

Following the tips and instructions, life with a newborn proved to be under control. Every day, I had a penciled-in blueprint of when baby would be awake, get hungry, and then take a nap. For us, it meant we'd eat, play, and then sleep—mostly uncompromising, in that order—about every three hours. This pattern allowed me to plan my time—trips to the market, the mall, the park, and anywhere else we wanted to go were all "scheduled" around when my girl would be awake, hungry, or sleepy.

If I had to drive across town for an appointment, I'd schedule it for a time when I knew I could comfortably feed her at home, load her in the car, and allow her to sleep in her seat during the long drive during a time that she'd be sleeping anyway. How do you think I managed to accomplish holiday shopping with long rides and multiple stops when my daughter was just two months old? I timed my life around her feed/play/sleep patterns. I felt organized, in control, and happy.

Establishing a schedule isn't easy, but no baby's going to teach herself how to do it. Training a baby means you must make a choice to do it and then *actually do what is necessary* with unwavering consistency. (You are a CEO now, remember?) Training a baby to get on schedule tests your ability to be a good leader for yourself and your child. It requires things like gently nudging your baby to wake up if she's sleeping "off-schedule," saying no thank you to visitors if they ask to come over during a time that's not conducive to your schedule-training, and perhaps syncing your daily timeline with your baby's needs in the name of setting a predictable schedule. (Yes, it's okay to nudge your baby awake if duty calls to train her on track! Don't be a wuss about it . . .) Obviously, there are exceptions, off days, and times of total chaos when there's no other choice but to call it all a loss and start fresh the next morning, but if you stay committed to creating a schedule within the first few months, the big payoff is worth it for your sanity and baby's health.

Setting daily schedules for baby is the only way to organize your time and days—it's also the only way a baby is going to learn the difference between her days and nights (which will then allow you time to rest and eventually proceed with normal life). Time is every mother's most precious commodity, so we must learn how to manipulate it early on . . . and make sure any childcare provider or family member helping you makes the effort to stick to your schedule, too! An organized baby is a happy baby; a happy baby makes a mom ecstatic, more capable, less stressed, positively focused, and in control. Once everyone's feeling good, it sets a fabulous precedent for looking good.

FAB tip! On Finding Childcare . . .

Even if you have family close by, start looking for childcare options that you can call on in random events of need right around the time your baby is one month old to ease your mind and prepare for the unexpected. Referrals always work best (whom did your friend use who lives in the area?), but you can also find tons of options through sitter or nanny agencies online that prescreen and background-check applicants before you even meet them. Be informed, be aware, and be cautious about whom you seek to watch your baby. When interviewing, heed the following tips:

1) Meet at a public place (rather than your home . . . everyone loves coffee).

2) Inform the applicant that you'd like to do a background check.

3) Be sure to ask if the applicant has any medical conditions that would be concerning should they be entrusted with your baby (do they suffer from seizures, etc.).

4) Ask if they are able to provide you with an all-clear note from their medical provider, saying they are fit and able to watch a baby.

5) Obtain referrals from previous employers (and call them!).

6) Open a conversation about "what-if" scenarios and how they'd handle it and discuss social media guidelines and habits (no scrolling Facebook while watching baby, no posting pictures of your baby on their Instagram account).

7) Educate yourself about early child brain development (reading, talking, singing to babies) and then instruct your childcare provider so they may extend and continue your efforts when you're not there.

8) Listen to your inner gut—it will speak to you in ways you never thought possible when it comes to finding childcare.

Most important: Bring your baby so the childcare provider can meet him or her. It's the only way to gauge how the caregiver connects with babies and if/how your baby will take to this new person!

CHAPTER 5

YOUR BIRTH BODY

inally! The part you've been waiting for! How to get that body rockin' again? Remember, I'm not going to get into details about why you'll want so many cold maxi-pads or whether there's such a thing as using that perineam spray bottle too much down there (there's not, by the way). Talk to your doctors and nurses about how to *medically* help heal your body (pain killers to lessen the shock of a C-section or Kegel exercises to strengthen your pelvic floor again). Your muscles will be sore and your body will probably not feel like your own anymore, but it will soon.

Since the purpose of this book is to foster resilience, I'll start with the tip that proved the most powerful, most liberating, and most effective for bouncing my body back fast after having my babies. It's also the tip that's going to cause a whole lot of ruckus for anyone who reads this book (and also for some who don't ever open this book). You might not like it, but I promised unfiltered honesty about what worked for me, so here it comes . . .

Shut Down the Milk Factory.

Yes, you're understanding this heading exactly as I mean it: opt out of breastfeeding if that's where your head is at. I know what you're thinking. *This is reckless. What new mother opts out of nursing a newborn? Breast milk is best. Is this another smack-talking war over nursing in public?* The answers to all those questions are: No it's not; This one; Yes it absolutely is; and No. Ask any new mom what her most tiresome, all-encompassing, and challenging task is during the first few months and, if she's like most of the women I've known through all walks of life and run into online, she will most likely tell you that nursing takes its toll in a mental, physical, and emotional way that no one ever warned her about.

Remember what I said at the very beginning of this no-frills journey together? All I can share are the choices that worked for me. Here's my truth that might be painful for some to believe: *Opting out of nursing allowed me to feel physically independent, free of pain, and exponentially less exhausted in those early days of motherhood compared to most of my peers who took the traditional route and nursed.*

Ditching nursing from Day One bounced me back fast, mind, body, and spirit. I do respect and honor women who choose to nurse (most of my friends have or do, and they're fabulous moms who have also bounced back!), and . . . breast milk is best! But opting out for me, twice in two years, set me on a most happy, confident, and productive track as a new mother.

You want personal? Okay. The reason I did not breastfeed either of my babies is that I simply was too freaked out to try it. I had no medical reason to give credit to my choice to formula-feed; I just feared the process of the alternative. The image of a mother holding her baby to her breast is the most natural thing in the world, and yet it absolutely scared me to death. Maybe I was immature? Maybe this fear was a result of how I was a formula-fed babe back in the late 1970s? We live in a breastfeed-or-defend-yourself-to-the-death society these days, but being honest with myself against all modern popular perception has made me into the kind of self-assured, deci-sion-making parent that I am proud to now be. Those who aren't afraid to make their own choices can rule the world.

It all started during my first pregnancy when my girlfriends asked me: why haven't you registered for nursing pads, detachable-strap bras, and nipple creams? Answer: I just couldn't picture myself doing all those things that breastfeeding moms do. I made the deci-sion to opt out practically the day I found out I was expecting. I half-considered nursing as my due date approached, mainly because of the pressure that exists to do it and the minimal educa-tion I got about the benefits for mom and baby prior to having the baby. Finally, I asked my husband (the pediatric surgeon), "Are you going to flip out if I don't nurse? Am I being stupid about this?" He (and his ten-plus years of medical school and specialty surgeon training) shrugged, "No. It's your choice." And it *was* my choice.

Simultaneously, my most incredible pediatrician I'd selected urged me to rethink my grand plan just before baby was born. The top-notch nurses tending to me the day after delivery were relent-less in educating me about the benefits of breast milk and tried to get me to change my mind. I smiled, resisted, and respectfully shut them down as politely as I could. (This rebel attitude coming from the same woman who's been bossing you to listen to your doctors and nurses. Ironic, I know.) The day after delivery, I was convinced to try pumping thanks to them selling me on the magical, nutritious power of colostrum (Liquid Gold, as it's known in maternity circles).

My patience for pumping lasted exactly eight days. I didn't produce much milk anyway (maybe because of my stressed-out, temporary high blood pressure issues postbirth the first time around) and ended up having to mix my unicorn-made Liquid Gold with store-bought formula to fill my new daughter's tiny belly . . . because, the point really is to feed a child so they can grow, whether it's exclusive breast milk or exclusive formula. (Exclusively feeding limited breast milk, without satisfying your baby's belly, is pointless if your child is screaming out of hunger.)

Despite the revelation of wow-look-at-what-my-body-can-produce thing, pumping was painful, annoying, exhausting, and genuinely draining me physically and emotionally every two hours on the dot. *I cannot go on like this and be normal or happy*, I remember agonizing. After those eight days, I shut down the milk factory. No guilt, no looking back, no regrets to bum me out. Exclusive formula feeding it was.

I repeated my pumping pattern for my second-born daughter a year and a half later in an effort to provide each newborn with identical care. But dealing with the physical effects of producing more milk than the first time, unexpected engorgement, leaking breasts, pumping, and feeding and handling a newborn were even more painful and challenging with another young child in the house, and it was too much. All I remember that first week after my second daughter was born was the piercing pain of milk exploding against my boobs from the inside out and panic about how I was going to overcome the physical torture to also take care of my older daughter (who was a year and a half at this time).

Why am I putting myself through this? Screw it. I have two daughters to take care of now, and if I can't give them a capable, able-bodied, and happy version of myself, then we're all going to crash and burn fast. After exactly eight days again, I happily shut down my own milk production. It was tougher to do this time around, but I was relentless. I used all kinds of desperate methods, including an experiment of lining my bra with fresh, frozen cabbage leaves for three days straight (replacing the wilted leaves with new cold leaves about every hour—I dare you to look this hysterical and fascinating method up online and yes, it worked for me). God bless my husband for those extra trips to the produce section. Exclusive formula-feeding it was again. Guess what: life with baby—and my toddler—got easy really fast.

Here are immediate perks I found to be true by bottle-feeding:

☺ *You know exactly how much milk baby's getting.*
Because you know how much milk is being sucked down, you're also going to have an accurate gauge on how much time you'll have before needing to do the next feeding. Meaning, you're going to know that baby's tummy is totally full (and will remain that way) for the next two to three hours at least, which means you can then put baby in her car seat and run an errand knowing that you're most likely not going to get stuck having to feed her in another hour. While breast-feeding moms often nurse every one to two hours in the beginning (assuming the baby fills her tummy each session, which you honestly don't know since you can't see the breast milk coming out like you can with a bottle), formula-feeding

moms often provide a bottle every three to four hours (since formula is less watery than breast milk). Take my word for it, three to four hours between feedings is *magic.*

☺ *Dad, friends, and family can help feed . . . no problem.*
Find me a mom who doesn't yearn for a break once a day—or in the middle of night—from feeding her precious new child and I will call major B.S. on you. Doing anything over and over again in a nonstop cycle has its mental and emotional challenges, even if the activity is something so sweet as feeding a newborn. With breastfeeding, you're stuck—you're the only one who can do it. With bottle-feeding, your world opens up. *Why, yes, mother-in-law—absolutely you can feed her! Oh darling husband—thank you for taking one of the night shifts so I might be able to rest to feel a bit more like a human the following day!* Bottle-feeding is smart, and don't let anyone tell you differently.

☺ *Your nipples won't bleed.*
This is not a scare mechanism. While many moms nurse easily and without drama (my own sister being one of them), many also come *this close* to their whole nipple practically falling off because of problems involving latching, sucking, chaffing, and all sorts of other things that I won't get into. Google it if you need to know details. I just knew I didn't want any part of that wicked possibility . . .

☺ *You don't feel as tired.*
The biological process to produce breast milk taxes and depletes the body, do not underestimate that. Breast-feeding

can zap you day after day, week after week, month after month, because you're literally making food to sustain another human being. I will never deny that creating breast milk is one of life's most incredible miracles, but let's not hide how much that miracle can truly exhaust a new mother to the point of near-delusional existence in today's demanding times. True, many moms attest their baby weight pretty much "fell off" while they nursed, but I also have an equal number of nursing friends who call a crock of you-know-what on that marketing myth, too.

☺ *You won't have that "when should I wean and how to do it" drama.*
Although many moms don't have any issues weaning or flip-flopping between bottle and breast, many do. And, if you've ever known a mom with a baby who won't take any kind bottle on account of wanting a breast (rightfully so, because that's the only thing they've had since birth), you'll know that it can be a most frustrating, stressful, confusing, and disappointing issue to deal with.

☺ *You feel physically similar to your prebaby self—except now you have a baby.*
This reality happens on account of not feeling as fatigued, not having scabbed and scarred nipples, not having three-inch puddles of milk staining your bras and blouses for all to see. (Obviously, you're still tired from broken sleep and night feedings, but it's not as intense because you're not producing milk.) Your body becomes yours again, which is major in the world of a new mom. Reclaiming your

physical autonomy instantly makes you feel more capable and organized.

Do breast-feeding moms have no choice but to be in unending pain and a hot mess? Hell no! My own sister still doesn't understand how I skipped out on nursing—she didn't experience any drama or negativity with breast-feeding that affected her day-to-day life. Which leads me to say, in special print, on the record:

If you've dreamed of nursing your baby, and it works for you, then do it! Just don't complain about it to the point that it drags you down, should it get tough.

The main reason I'm pegging formula feeding as a cornerstone of bouncing back is that the majority of complaints I've heard about new motherhood revolve around nursing challenges. Check out any new mom Facebook group and you'll see what I mean in about five seconds. What drives me crazy, online and in real life, is when I see smart, capable, and highly educated women struggling, crying, stressed, and practically tearing their hair out over not producing enough milk, their babies not latching on, living in extreme physical pain (that bleeding nipple thing again), or just not enjoying nursing to the point that it's making them depressed, frustrated, and panicked.

These same women often continue to lament in a torturous state, begging, "What should I do?!" and "How can I solve this problem, fellow mamas?!" for the sake of trying to breast-feed exclusively for the "benefits." What to do? *Either figure out how to solve the problem without drama or stop breast-feeding altogether.* Nobody reaps any benefits whatsoever from breast-feeding if it's agonizing to mom, baby, or both at the same time, mentally, emotionally, or physically.

For working moms, breast-feeding can be tumultuous. For starters, returning to work when baby is just a few months (or weeks) old can be very stressful itself. I get it—working moms want to do right by their babies, especially because they're not at home all day. Making milk is taxing on the body, and no new mom who is working full-time should have to feel like she's obligated to be four different women in one just to give her baby breast milk. Pumping at work can be tricky (although many workplaces are making progress, and there are newer and more discreet pumps on the market these days), but why put yourself through the strain and anxiety to do it all? Being overextended will most certainly affect your family in a negative way, even if you are trying to provide breast milk.

Stress can prevent a woman's body from producing enough breast milk in the first place, which then can (wrongly) make any new working mom feel inadequate. Feeling guilty for working or not producing enough milk can quickly spin into an uncontrollable and intense struggle between emotions, stress, time management, and mental clarity. Is it worth all the drama? I have a friend who spun herself into a tizzy because she wasn't producing enough milk to satisfy her baby . . . yet she refused to give up breast-feeding because it wasn't in her plan. Modern women know the importance of giving ourselves breaks, so give one to yourself in the breast-feeding department if it's only making you feel bad. Life comes along when you're making other plans, remember?

The American College of Obstetrics and Gynecology (ACOG) cites, "Women who experience breastfeeding difficulties are at higher risk of postpartum depression and should be screened, treated, and referred appropriately." I don't relay these words with any kind of sleazy intention to skew facts or mislead you to believe that breast-feeding directly leads to postpartum depression. But read the words *at higher risk* associated with breast-feeding difficulties. If you start experiencing major issues with breast-feeding that take you down an emotional, mental, or physical spiral to a dark, self-doubting place you can't seem to pull yourself out of, then why not nip it all in the bud and save yourself and your baby unnecessary trauma?

Make no mistake, I'm not disputing that breast milk is an incomparable living food. There's a reason the American Academy of Pediatrics recommends breast milk for the first year. However, formulas approved by the Food and Drug Administration also contain sufficient nutrients for baby's growth and development; all formulas sold in the United States are perfectly safe and must adhere to the Infant Formula Act, which was developed to safeguard formula manufacturing and nutritional health of infants. A 2014 study published by the *Social Science & Medicine* journal determined that there was not a marked difference in child development (body mass index, obesity, asthma, hyperactivity, parental attachment, behavior compliance, achievement in vocabulary, reading recognition, math ability, intelligence, and scholastic competence) when comparing formula-fed babies with their breast-fed siblings . . . leading us to believe that genetics determines an awful lot more than breast milk when it comes to growing babies.

Additionally, the ACOG issued an updated statement on breast-feeding versus bottle feeding as of January 2016, citing that obstetrician–gynecologists and other obstetric care providers "should support each woman's informed decision about whether to initiate or continue breastfeeding, recognizing that she is uniquely qualified to decide whether exclusive breastfeeding, mixed feeding, or formula feeding is optimal for her and her infant." Educate yourself about the benefits and costs, but don't be afraid to make choices that you can feel fully comfortable with. Muster up the courage to do what feels right for you, your body, and your baby. It's okay to make a choice that goes against the popular, all-natural grain as long as you're responsible and heed the advice of credible, expert authorities about providing the alternative choice.

For a while, I kept my bottle-feeding a secret from many of the high profile parenting groups I was involved with because, if you don't breast-feed in Los Angeles, then you're cheating! When mom-friends of mine would talk about nursing challenges or commiserate about how much they wished their nursing days to be over, I'd just stay quiet that. I'd worry whether my dirty secret would be found out. (Was my bottle-fed baby developing differently? No.) It wasn't until years later that I admitted my secret to Cheryl Petran, CEO and owner of the famous nursing support mecca The Pump Station & Nurtury in Santa Monica, California.

To my surprise, Cheryl laughed at me and responded with, "Judgment? No, no judgment here!" Cheryl later went on the record for one of my CBS television news segments that addressed guilt and formula-feeding moms, saying, "Whether she is unable to or simply making the choice not to breastfeed, no mother should be harboring any feelings of guilt . . . it serves no purpose for the mother or the child in terms of health, well-being, and attachment." I still smile whenever I think of Cheryl's words—all this wisdom coming from a woman whose beliefs and livelihood revolve around breast-feeding babies. And here I thought she'd wipe me off her friend list.

Since then, a few other deep thoughts have struck me: some women get night nurses or full-time nannies from the day their babies are born and hire help for a variety of duties that, like breast-feeding, are known to encourage mother/child bonding—nap rituals, diaper changing, bath time, and play time. Some women return to high-powered jobs just days or weeks after birth and entrust their babies to someone else's primary care. Some new moms move out of their own house to live with their parents (without their spouses) to score free round-the-clock assistance. Moms who make those kinds of choices are not judged nearly as much as nonnursing moms, so I'd be damned if I was going to fear being judged for staying home, not hiring a nanny, and opting to give my baby an FDA-approved alternative to breast milk.

In a complicated world where new moms are encouraged to make all sorts of choices to maintain emotional stability and physical health, know that opting out of breast-feeding also falls under that same "self-care" canopy. Yes, you can still bond with your baby without using your boobs (I did with both my girls . . . playing, talking, cuddling, and singing counts as bonding, too). Yes, your baby's brain will develop just fine if he is fed with infant formula (assuming he is healthy at birth). Yes, your child can still go to Harvard even if she was fed with a bottle. And no, no one ever asks whether your kid was nursed on college admission applications or the first day of kindergarten (except maybe that condescending mom who lives down the street . . . but screw her).

In the spirit of fair and balanced reporting here, I will repeat: my sister nursed both of her babies for about six months each, and she bounced back fast! What was the key to her success? 1) She really wanted to nurse, 2) nursing came fairly easily without major issues, and 3) she stopped nursing when her milk production drastically changed—that's it. Rather than mentally and physically fighting her own body, putting herself through the emotional torment of "why aren't I producing more?" and trying all kinds of hokey-pokey potions and exercises to make more milk, she instead gave herself intelligent permission to accept her body's rhythm and let her boobies shut down, guilt free. There's honor in working hard to finish a job the way you first envision it, but there's also practical value for all parties involved by just letting things be. The last thing a baby needs is a stressed-out mom, especially if that stress is tied to feeding the baby.

My newborn days and first years of motherhood, both times, were not challenging, difficult, painful, or hazy; they were *fun and fulfilling*. I remember feeling tired, but never completely depleted and exhausted, and I'm absolutely sure it's because I formula-fed my girls. My daughters are both healthy, and, as of this writing, all development is right on track. (Aha, the formula worked!) Choosing something so unconventional within my immediate parenting surroundings tapped into a powerful confidence I didn't know I had. That confidence has shaped my resilience as a mother to this day and has positively affected my kids (as babies and beyond). Newborns need moms who take charge for every-one's greater good more than they need our actual boobs. If you ain't feelin' the breast-feeding or if it's causing you major stress, then bounce fast—because the bottle makes everything easier, baby.

(I say that with genuine admiration and respect for the nursing moms who tirelessly really do enjoy it without any complaint.)

3 Fixes for Nursing Without Drama

From Dr. Tanya Altmann, mom, pediatrician, founder of Calabasas Pediatrics & author of What to Feed Your Baby

I first met Dr. Tanya at a Los Angeles blogger event back in 2013. She's impressively accomplished and celebrated in pediatric medicine, and we seemed to immediately click (go UCLA Bruins)—she also happens to be absolutely down-to-earth with her parenting expertise. When I told her about my choice to formula-feed, she didn't agree with me, but she understood and supported where I was coming from as a friend. Here are her tips for nursing while keeping nipple drama at bay . . .

1. **Ask for help!** Although breast-feeding is natural, most babies aren't born experts. It may take days or weeks for a newborn to catch on. Often, just one meeting with a lactation consultant can make a world of difference for long-term breast-feeding success.
2. **No pain allowed**. Breast-feeding can feel a little weird, like tugging at your breast, but it shouldn't hurt. If you're having pain, it's most likely that your baby isn't latching on properly, so take her off and try again or ask for help obtaining the perfect fish-lip latch position.
3. **Introduce a bottle**. Once breast-feeding is well established, usually by three or four weeks of age, pump and offer your baby a bottle once a day; this is a great way for Dad or a caretaker to bond with the baby. It will also teach (and

remind) baby how to drink from a bottle for if/when you return to work . . . or if you ever want to leave baby and go out! (Note: Don't be afraid of nipple confusion! If your baby is solidly nursing, offering a bottle will not confuse her!)

Fake It? Make It!

Let's just go ahead and call this section Showbiz Mom 101. What, you didn't know that show business and motherhood are pretty much the same things? They are. I know from experience, along with so many of my television news reporter friends who tirelessly work often-unreasonable hours in the field at fast-paced speeds that would exhaust any new mom. Oh, but wait! Those reporter friends of mine who look good and speak clearly and appear perfectly in order on your local channel *are also new moms*. How do they do it? How do *we* do it? We fake it when duty calls. Same rules apply to motherhood, especially when it comes to looking good from the outside the months following delivery.

I'll never forget how fabulous my friend, anchor and reporter Courtney Friel from Los Angeles' KTLA news, looked just a few weeks after delivering her second child. Courtney invited a bunch of families over for her birthday, so I packed up my people and headed over with my husband—my younger daughter was a little over a month old. I was feelin' pretty good (hey, I know how to fake it); I wore a jumper and some silver flat sandals. We arrived and rang the doorbell. Courtney answered the door in full-on makeup, chandelier earrings, a fitted floral tank dress, and platform shoes that had me feeling instantly dumpy in my flats. "Oh my gosh . . .

you look amazing!" the words flew out of my mouth before I even said hello decently. Her face lit up and she announced, "I'm a FAB mom!" standing there in the doorway. I think of that moment every time I get ready for a party to this day.

Here's the thing about show business: a lot of it is about faking how fabulous you can look and fooling others to believe you're more pulled together than you actually might feel. We all know about airbrushing in magazines, but how about employing a bit of airbrushing for real-life, in-person encounters for those first three months after you pop a baby out of your body? Yes, it's possible and recommended (if you're talking to me, anyway). You might not feel good, you might not look your best, but by hot damn you can fake it just as good as anyone else and fool them all. And no one will be the wiser.

Where to start? With the midsection, of course. If you were paying attention back in 2013, Kate Middleton made a splashing, news-making debut right after she gave birth to Britain's first royal baby in recent years, Prince George. You might recall how practically every news outlet and parenting blog was praising Duchess Kate for showing what a real woman looked like postbirth—by stepping outside the hospital with what looked like a five-month pregnant belly under her dress. *Yes! That is what a brand new mom's midsection really looks like, folks! Way to be real.* Don't be shocked if you still look several months pregnant when your beautiful baby is swaddled right next to you on Day 3, postdelivery. That's all fine and natural, and we can all know and own the truth, but this book is about bouncing back. So, how to fool everyone that you're a freak of nature in the body department after having a baby? Get yourself a postpartum wrap, pronto.

About two weeks after delivering my second daughter back in March 2012, I went to a celebrity shopping event to launch maternity businesswoman Rosie Pope's new clothing line Rosie Pope Maternity. Physically, I felt good and was itching to get out of the house a bit (the birth of a second or third baby always seems to be much more manageable). I was interested to see this new, chic clothing line up close, mostly because I was a huge fan of Rosie. I additionally wanted to challenge myself to see if I could fool anyone, myself included, about how I'd had a baby just two weeks prior. (Call that a desperate postpartum ego trip.) I tightened my tummy wrap that I'd been wearing 24/7 since the day after my recent delivery and drove the full hour to Santa Monica's Montana Boulevard. Truth be told, I couldn't quite move my body because the taut was so tight. It was like my core was in a neck brace from hell . . . you get me?

I parked my car, stepped out in my four-inch high-heeled black boots, made sure my blouse was covering my covert mommy-girdle, and walked into the bright, white store. I made my way through racks of stunning silhouettes—dresses, pants, skirts, and tops. A part of me was pissed I wasn't pregnant anymore; the clothes were stunning! Model and actress Molly Simms was there, pregnant with her first child, taking pictures for press with television personality and famous mother of four Brooke Burke-Charvet (at this time, Brooke was still cohost of ABC's *Dancing with the Stars*). I saw Brooke standing across the room, and a shock hit me. *OMG! The tummy wrap I'm wearing is part of Brooke's Baboosh Body line for postbaby compression! I am wearing HER product!*

Should I tell her? Should I run up and lift up my shirt? As the event went on, I eventually found myself standing in a group with her, Molly, and a bunch of mom bloggers making awkward conversation. I wanted to shout, "Brooke! I'm wearing your belly wrap right now and I just had a baby not even two weeks ago and I feel great and no one here believes that I just had a baby and did I mention I feel great and this is soooooo amazing!!!" But, I didn't . . . because that would've been weird and I did not want anyone calling security on an aggressive crazy lady who just had a baby, lifting up her blouse and showing off her tummy wrap for all to see. But man, did I feel good that night because of that corset around my core. I faked it and felt like I'd made it . . . and I've been shouting the benefits of committing to postpartum wraps ever since.

So, here's your one and only list of what you need to fake your way to fabulousness, from the outside in, during the early weeks and months after having a baby:

🙂 *Postpartum Tummy Wrap*
There are a ton of brands available. All you need to do is pick one and commit to wearing it. (I personally think Belly Bandit has the biggest variety of options these days to tackle a wide variety of pregnancy and postpartum needs for the whole body.) Thanks to your sweet baby being in your belly and shoving your bladder to one side and your stomach all the way up your esophagus, the inside of your midsection is going to feel like a loosey-goosey hot mess after delivery. A postpartum tummy wrap made me feel more comfortable and should be worn starting one to two days after delivery and continue for about six to eight weeks following birth. I wore mine for about forty days (as suggested by Brooke Burke-Charvet), morning and night (I did not take it off, except to wash it and to shower), and yes, it shrunk my belly within weeks. For my first birth, my waist measured 40 inches before delivery, 36 inches just after delivery, and 30 inches five weeks postpartum—that's

a loss of 10 inches in just over a month! If you wear them right (very, very tight, like a girdle), postpartum wraps are also medically recognized to help healing, minimize water retention, and encourage organs to shrink back to normal size and make you feel optimally supported in the back and core from the inside out. Added bonus? They make you look slimmer, faster, on the outside, too.

☺ *Compression Tank Tops and Leggings*
These babies weren't really around right after I had my babes, but I wish they were (because yeah, I wear them now). Not only will the compression material in the tank make you feel extrasupported around the core, but the specialized density of fabric offering 360-degree support around your legs will also help with water retention and any budding varicose veins. I always felt more capable in reinforced, stretchy gear around the house while taking care of a newborn. And it's all stretchy, so you still feel comfortable enough to lie down and sneak in that nap when baby's sleeping. (Again, Belly Bandit offers these.)

☺ *Sneakers*
Just as pliable leggings allow you to do the manual labor that a baby requires while still feeling comfortable (rocking her, holding her, tossing a load of soiled onesies in the washing machine), sneakers are a must-wear during those early days. Something that surprised me after birth was that my body felt floppy and sore. I'm not talking about being floppy and sore "down there" (although you will be, if you don't have a C-section); I'm talking about

all-around fatigue and dull pain through my muscles, in my bones, and at my joints. No matter how you give birth, your body will go through a lot to get that baby out. Do yourself a favor and wear shoes that will help your entire physical self. Sneakers support your back, your legs, your core so that you can move effectively and pain-free . . . which will then support your mind and spirit in the long run and get you back into your cute strappy shoes soon enough.

☺ Tinted dry shampoo

Even though your baby will most likely sleep a lot (most newborns do), you will somehow not be able to take a shower like you used to. Every mom I know looks back at her newborn days and says, "Why couldn't I take a shower with a newborn in the house? They just lay there and barely moved!" It's a question none of us can answer, so I won't try to make sense of it here. However, your hair will get dirty . . . and you may or may not feel like washing it. Also, your hair might certainly fall out (doctors estimate that 30 to 50 percent of women have significant hair loss postpartum thanks to natural hormone depletions and readjustments that follow birthing a baby). On top of all this, you might not be able to get those gray hairs covered up like you did before baby. Get yourself some dry shampoo that has a color tint to match your hair and you'll be all set to fool everyone that you wash your hair, color your roots, and have zero hair loss (thanks to the tinted color clinging to your thinning hairline and scalp).

Self-Tanning Lotion & Bronzer

Before you accuse me of resurrecting the 1995 Malibu Barbie look, listen to this: a bronzed body automatically appears about ten pounds thinner. (Why do you think I still bother to slather that brown, self-tanning lotion on my arms every time I wear a sleeveless top on television?) What else makes you feel perky and alive from the outside? A sun-kissed face. Grab yourself some bronzing powder and brush it on your cheeks, chin, forehead, and nose à la Jennifer Lopez. The visual trick of having a warm glow makes you look a bit more svelte and awake—a sneaky trick that all on-camera personalities and former pageant girls know to be effective. (Hey, I once won the swimsuit competition at the Miss California pageant partially thanks to some strategic shadowing around the abs . . . just sayin'. Please don't take away my crown.) If the bronzing makes you look more toned before babies, it'll work just the same after babies, too. So why not use it?

Yes, I realize this list might come off as extremely shallow (we're smarter than this!), but if you manage to fool others into perceiving how "fabulous" you look on the outside so soon after having a baby, you also prompt yourself to feel better from the inside. Call it a jacked-up circumstance of impossible and wrongly ingrained social standards, but it is what it is: the old "if you look good, you feel good" trick strikes again.

3 Fixes for Dressing the After-Baby Bod

From Orly Shani, mom, designer of TUC+WES by Orly Shani, DIY & style expert, TV host

Fun fact! I first met Orly when we briefly worked together as on-camera experts for Hallmark Channel's *Home & Family* show in 2013. Because her sitter flaked on a day she was working on set, she brought her then-baby boy with her and handled the work day like a momboss. I had immediate admiration and affection for her feisty problem-solving, bounce-through-this skills. Not to mention, she's a flippin' talented designer. Orly's tips on dressing the postbump bod . . .

1. **Dress your *new* figure.** Some women bounce right back to their prebaby body and can wear the same wardrobe as before, but for others, that's not the case. There can be new lumps and bumps to contend with; some fun, and some not so much. Reassess your new figure and give it some love with a few fab choices to highlight this new body best. Look at photos of celebrities who have a similar body and get ideas . . . or, as I like to say: hijack that stylist!

2. **Get new undergarments!** Boobs can completely disappear after babies (if you nurse), so new bras are a must. I bought sexy, lace bralettes that looked cute with my nonboobs along with a few insanely padded, va-va-va-voom bras! Having both made me feel confident in my new body.

3. **Do your makeup . . .** Okay, maybe this doesn't seem easy for everyone, but a little eyelash-curler, undereye concealer,

126

blush, and lipstick always makes me feel like a new woman! I hated seeing myself as that frazzled new mom at the market. Five minutes of love in the morning makes me feel more like myself all day long . . . and, frankly, makes me a whole lot more fun to be around. (No need for Kardashian level contouring; little dabs will do.)

Faking your way to looking good is savvy, but I'm guessing you want to actually get yourself looking good, too. Best way to start the process is to take that baby of yours on a walk in the stroller, ASAP (given that it's not raining, snowing, or sweltering hot outside). As soon as your doctor gives you a go-ahead to start moving around, go for it. My maiden solo stroller voyage with Baby #1 happened at exactly the one-month postpartum mark. I loaded my little gal and rolled down our street while having mild panics about how a bee kept circling us as we walked—I remember swatting and swinging my arms in a way that had passers-by wondering why I was so paranoid; it was quite a scene.

Almost every day, I'd make a point to take her on a fifteen-minute walk after I fed her so that I could exercise, she could look around at the world, and we could both get some fresh air. It was physically good for both of us. Sometimes, I'd even stop the stroller and do some squats (for my thighs and butt) if no one was around. Turns out, this kind of new mom exercise with a stroller is known as Fit4Mom (formerly called Stroller Strides) and was founded by a fantastic L.A. woman by the name of Lisa Druxman—look them up to find one offered in an area near you. Or just take your baby out for a few fifteen-minute walks per day and do pushups on the curb to get started on your own.

You know what else makes your arms and body extrasvelte after having a baby? Not depending on one of those trendy baby carriers that everyone's into. I know, you have a friend who swears by its ability to make life hands-free with a newborn. Here are a few things that everyone seems to overlook: 1) If you're constantly carrying a baby around effortlessly, your arms and upper body will never get any kind of workout, 2) Your baby might get accustomed to automatically being stuck to you at all times and start throwing major fits should you pull him off and away from your body for any reason (I've known this to happen to several friends of mine), which makes life as a new mom that much harder, and 3) It's pretty much inevitable that you'll soon feel like you're pregnant again, carrying a full load in front of you at all times, so why would you want to live in a constant state that you're not obligated to? Use a baby carrier few and far between—when you absolutely need it for traveling, if you're heading to Disneyland and have no desire to push a stroller, or if it's the last resort for getting your babe to stop crying so you can grocery shop in peace.

All frivolity about pageant tricks and tummy girdles aside, a true and lasting bounceback thoroughly depends on your ability to clearly see and love the new you with some sneaky tricks thrown in for added laughs—even if this "new you" is shaped differently from before baby came along. What's a freaky and fabulous way to do this? Open your underwear drawer.

Get Your Panties On . . .

If opting out of nursing is the most controversial tip in this book, then this next task I'm adding to your list may be considered the most absurd. Ready for it?

Walk around in only your underwear at home for the first month.
(Curtains and blinds closed, of course.)

That's right, during the previously suggested, self-induced thirty-day lockdown of newborn swaddling and scheduling, I hereby order you to wear a wardrobe exclusively of panties and camisoles. (No, I'm not a pervert.) Who knew that spending full days pretty much naked would be my solution to so many changes and uncertainties during that first month with baby? No shame, no excuses, no regard for what anyone else might think. This ridiculous habit did wonders for my postpartum body confidence and I'm convinced it will for you, too. (No, I'm not drunk as I write this.)

I pulled this pretty panty trick after the births of both my daughters, and I recommend it to any new mom willing to try and trust the process. This offbeat experiment came to fruition right after the birth of Baby #1 because of three major circumstances crashing together at the same time: 1) It was crazy hot outside (late September in Los Angeles), and we wanted to save money on air conditioning bills, 2) I was just too damn lazy to get dressed for the sake of tending to a newborn in my home that no one could see into from the outside, and 3) I was absolutely and unreasonably petrified of becoming "frumpy" after having a baby. (Let's just say the third reason really propelled my spirit . . .)

As I spilled at the beginning of this book, all random tales I'd heard about motherhood prior to having a baby myself pointed to how moms—especially new moms—never have energy to do anything associated with their former life, including activities involving cute underwear. The concept of being a mom meant trading all sexy underthings for a bunch of baby junk decked with dorky designs. Not to mention, everyone kept telling me to run out and buy as many granny panties as I could prior to having my baby. *Woohoo. Let the wild fun begin. New Mom = Boring Underwear = Boring Life.* All this wisdom was according to my personal book of ignorance back then, so I thought, *Why not fight it?*

Like a real genius (a really dumb genius), I refused to buy any kind of high-waist underwear for postbirth comfort just to prove everyone wrong about "needing" granny panties after delivery. I packed my low-rise (but almost full-bottomed cotton) panties complete with lace trims into my hospital bag and was smug about the thought of pulling them on and shocking all the nurses into commenting, "Wow, you sure know how to stay 'you' right after baby!"

The day after delivery, I was uncomfortable, immobile (thanks to that C-section slice), and helplessly stuck in those how-are-these-sanitary-and-legal mesh shorts that the hospital gives you after birth because I was too headstrong to buy comfortable high-waist beforehand. Keep in mind, that tender incision across my belly was ironically positioned in the exact same spot on my body where the lace trim from my low-rise panties I'd packed fit on my body (ouch, to say the least). Sagging, bloating, farting, aching, snipping, and scarring in places that should never be snipped or scarred . . . and now ugly undergarments made of mesh. So far, motherhood seemed like a real buzzkill.

I fell in love with my baby girl immediately, but the back of my ambitious mind was trying to solve the underwear dilemma right there in my hospital room. *How to keep frumpy away?* My scheming went into overdrive when I saw my reflection in my hospital room's fluorescent-lit bathroom mirror: I looked like a stuffed sausage in a hot pink tank top (that was just from the waist up). I then looked down at my legs: two stuffed sausages in flimsy shorts made of netting (with a maxi-pad stuck to the inside). I looked better when

I was pregnant. *How can I stop this shock and start feeling good about my postbaby bod?*

The realization that most new mothers have hit me right then: no matter how much or little weight you gain during pregnancy, your body will look, feel, and act differently after you have that baby, and it will affect you in some way. We can't help it. I looked at my reflection, and a quick and delirious solution came to me, standing on my two sausages: shock diminishes when you're exposed to something constantly. So . . .

If newborns could spend entire days in their underwear—their onesies—then so could I.
So I did.

Remember, this was all before the days of those recurring Instagram pictures from random half-naked women and digital campaigns from beauty brands that now feature women's sagging postpartum skin, wrinkly belly buttons in bikinis and C-section scars on display in the name of body confidence and mom-empowerment . . . but let me tell you, my trick worked. *Man, did it work.*

Since it was so warm outside when my first daughter was born, why not take care of her solely in my undies? Between feeding, rocking, changing, and wiping my newborn's butt, I spent ridiculous efforts resurrecting frilly robes, lace-trimmed camisoles, cropped tanks, push-up bras, boy-short panties (the kind that didn't irritate my C-section), and even threw on a few of my flowing lingerie baby-dolls (over my granny panties) for the kick of it. Yes, I also ordered some high-waist cotton panties in bold colors and prints. I was in my home, with my baby, in my new body, and I was adamant about doing what I pleased in only my underwear.

It was freeing in a most unexpected way. While my babe lay content in her rocker, I washed bottles, tossed in laundry loads, and cleaned my apartment in my undies. I ate bagels on the couch while watching bad reality shows, as she napped in her bassinet, in my undies. I held her and rocked her in my undies. I was half-naked, reading and singing to my new girl, with each of us in our onesies for about a month. You can imagine the scramble when the UPS guy rang the doorbell.

Once I got past certain inhibitions about the strangeness of it all (who the hell walks around in underwear all day?), the process proved to be most liberating on an extreme emotional and physical level. Constantly living life and seeing myself in a scanty wardrobe encouraged me to accept and feel better about my changed body. I *needed* to see my new body and all its unfamiliar new markings in full form—every day, all day— so that I could get *used* to it. Forging an honest and intimate relationship with that unexplained, vertical dark line down the center of my belly and my swelled tummy *desensitized* me. I quickly became conditioned *not to judge myself* every time I passed a mirror. I became unfazed by my body's changes because I saw myself in full form over and over again without relief—as opposed to just catching fleeting glimpses when I showered.

Within a few weeks, I found myself feeling comfortable, oddly inspired, and more like my before-baby self every day . . . which made me happier, more capable, and motivated as a parent. For starters, you realize that your baby will love you no matter how floppy your naked tummy might feel. I also figured, if I could commit to keeping appealing underwear and camisoles active and out of the back of my drawers while also learning to be comfortable in my new self, then washing my hair, wearing lipstick, and getting my energy back would follow quickly (it all did). The unexpected perk was that my husband seemed to be amused by it all, with raised eyebrows that questioned, "You spent all day in your underwear?" when he'd get home from work.

Accepting your body gets easier when you decide to form a friendship with it, flaws and all; the more you see it, the more you tend to like it. I also challenge you not to crack up at the ridiculousness of seeing yourself in the mirror, standing in cute underwear and holding a baby in your arms. Underwear-ing keeps things fun and funny during the mundane "newborn groundhog days" of sleeping, crying, feeding, changing, wiping, and repeating five times over until doing it all again the very next day. And the most satisfying thing that will most likely happen is that, one day when you least expect it, you'll catch your mostly naked body in the mirror as you dash to get another burp cloth and think, "You know what, I look pretty good." No, your body didn't change— your mind just did.

Turns out, requiring a new mom to be half-naked for an ongoing period of time might be beyond-empowering for babies, too. While skin-to-skin contact benefits parent and infant bonding minutes after birth (DNA and brain pathways are impacted by connectivity and separation between mothers and newborns, and skin-to-skin contact makes babies feel safe and secure—look it up if you're interested), who's to say that skin-to-skin benefits stop once you get the baby home? Granted, I've got no scientific research to back this up, but here's how I see it: extended skin-to-skin contact through the first few weeks, via a mom taking care of her infant in her underwear, certainly can't hurt.

My postpartum panty-palooza (after each of my baby girls, twice in two years) made me feel strong, happy, capable, and confident, regardless of how different I looked in my reflection. The more we commit to quickly *accepting our real selves* right after birth, the faster our bodies seem to bounce back . . . simply because we become more content and not bogged down with pointless pining about an extra pinch here or an additional roll there. Here's to getting seminaked every day, all day, for thirty days. Choose to love your body, even if you enlist attractive underwear to kick-start it. (And yes, I sometimes still rock the panty-raid for old time's sake—just don't come knockin' on my door for a show.)

Now, time for real matters of the heart . . .

FAB tip! On Getting Sleep

One thing remains constant when it comes to the body: make sure you get sleep. Although I've given direction (and will continue to give direction) about key things to think about or tasks to do once baby arrives, do not forget to find time to rest between the to-dos I'm suggesting. Finding time to lie down and close your eyes (even if it's just for a fifteen-minute power nap) trumps all other chores and minimissions I discuss throughout this book. I remember feeling dead tired some days and full of energy other days, and you'll most likely have your ups and downs, too.

In the very early days, I remember thinking, "I can't close my eyes, I have a baby to keep alive!" Remember this throughout your journey: if a newborn is secure and belted in a rocker or bassinet with no blankets on top of him, already fed, and/or content (e.g., not crying), then you are absolutely permitted to let yourself doze off on the couch while your babe stares at the ceiling or watches his melodic elephant mobile that your sister gave as a gift turn around and around. Newborns can't get into any trouble on their own—they can't even sit up! Taking brief snoozes while the baby is content (and preferably sleeping) is part of your job as a new mother, for self-care purposes. Don't skimp on the part of your job that is most important to keep you running and CEO-ing in the most productive way possible. You are in survival mode now—train yourself to cash in on spurts of sleep when opportunity strikes, even if you must bust out that light-blocking sleep mask I recommended you getting earlier to do it.

It's been said that functioning on sleep deprivation is similar to asking someone drunk to drive a car. And nobody—not baby, your spouse, or yourself—likes a drunk new mom.

CHAPTER 6
YOUR BIRTH HEART

Emotions run superhigh after having a baby. Blame our hormones, blame scattered skill sets for coping with change, blame that severe sleep deprivation that usually catches up with us around Day Five after delivery (which can make us sob our eyes out), or blame that our baby won't stop crying no matter what we try. That first week—hello, the first few weeks—might be a big blur. It's normal, be aware of it. You will have times of overpowering love and you will have times of overpowering what-the-hell-was-that. Your love life might change, evolve, diminish, flourish, and then confuse you all over again. What's the trick to keeping ebbs and flows of love and emotions moving in a positive direction? Your ability to adapt to change.

New Love with Your Spouse.

A baby will show you how much love you really have to give, and he will also teach you how much love can instantly change with those around you. As much as this pains me to admit, I really didn't like my husband right after having our first baby—if you read the letter for fathers, this isn't news. My husband tended to our daughter so phenomenally and compassionately, and really helped me before I could fully function (post-C-section). He was great working along-side my mom during baby's first days in our home. After that, I was pretty much irritated, constantly, for the following few weeks. (I still don't know why—I'm going to blame that nasty postpartum high blood pressure again.) I quickly discovered our love did not seem the same as before; it was suddenly different, unfamiliar, and confusing to me. If you find yourself having offbeat feelings or resentment toward your spouse after baby, don't fret. It happens to the best of us.

Throughout my first pregnancy, the few existing mom-friends I had back then warned me not to get too swept away in Babyland and ignore my husband once our baby arrived . . . but never did it cross my mind that I might feel like *he* was ignoring *me*! For the first few weeks after birth, I felt like I could count the number of times my husband looked at me on one hand. Keep in mind, we were still considered newlyweds at that point (had been blissfully married for only about one year), which made my once-solid faith about keeping a marriage hot and alive after baby plummet. Every single bit of his attention was on our daughter and, man, did it peeve me. As much as I adored our new baby, I admit to feeling a bit envious.

I'm not saying babies shouldn't get more attention than adults (they should, they're babies), but as someone who went through quite an ordeal to bring another person into this world, I started feeling very dispensable. *Now that she's had the baby . . . who needs her?* We enjoyed our early days of brand-new parenthood, but I soon felt like I didn't know my husband the same way I did before. Who *was* this person, and did he notice that *I* was also in the room? *How immature and selfish of me.* What mom gets huffy that her baby is sucking away all the attention from the other parent? That's crazy. Maybe the lack of normal sleep was getting to me, but everything felt so real—and I hated that I was feeling those kinds of things in the first place. *Is this when the honeymoon ends? Damn.* I quickly decided our before-baby bliss was not going to disappear without a fight.

I pulled the rip cord to restore balance in our marriage. My mind flashed to worse-case relationship scenarios that we've all read or heard about: if I passively chilled out and let our lack of quality interaction continue, two weeks would quickly turn into one month, which would then flash into one year, which would grow into two years, and so on and so on. I saw that glimpse of how easy it is to forget about yourself and your spouse once a newborn arrives, and I didn't like it one bit. There is a time to enjoy your new baby, but there is also a time to remind yourself that you and your husband were here *first*.

I'm not talking about having sex this early in the game (ouch— trust me, you're most likely not going to want to do anything down there for months); I'm simply talking about staying connected to each other on a PG-13 emotional level by chatting, holding hands, laughing, and relating to each other day in and day out (I mean, your doctor probably won't even give you the go-ahead to have sex before eight weeks after baby anyway).

In a panic, here's how I nipped the growing disdain-for-husband in the bud and conquered a marriage reset about a month after baby was born:

☺ *I shaved my legs.*

☺ *I brushed my hair. (I also brushed my teeth.)*

☺ *I put on (minimal) makeup so I looked decent when he came home.*

☺ *I threw on that cute shirt I hadn't worn since my before-pregnancy days.*

☺ *I reminded myself to smile more.*

☺ *I cooked a fresh dinner three nights in one week—instead of plopping down one of our frozen meals that I'd prepared prior to delivery.*

☺ *I popped open a bottle of wine (for both of us).*

☺ *I made it a point to cuddle up with my husband and coo at our baby, together.*

☺ *I reignited my silly habit of sneaking up behind him and squeezing his butt.*

☺ *I started conversations about things that had nothing to do with our child.*

☺ *I put on a (comfortable) piece of lingerie without any reason or expectation for action—which made both of us laugh out loud.*

☺ *I handwrote him a note detailing all the things I loved and admired about him.*

I committed to tackling these trivial tasks within a one-week period and checked them off my "list" as I did them. As dated and 1950s as this seems, these to-dos actually helped restore our connection. The love letter was most powerful: there's something surprisingly genuine and fulfilling, from both sides, about writing and reading thoughts and feelings on paper. (Or maybe I just found it cathartic because I like to write?) My trite to-dos renewed my own energy and got me enjoying my marriage again. I was relieved for us to feel like a couple once more, a team committed to our newborn, and this made our relationship better as we shifted from "newlyweds" to "new family."

The first celebrity couple I remember hearing about prioritizing their marriage before babies was former *E! News* host Giuliana Rancic and Bill Rancic. Back in 2013, Giuliana went on the record and said she puts her marriage before her baby. She got some heat for saying that, but I was nodding my head and saying "Yes, woman." And do you remember that big hubbub about television host and model Chrissy Teigen and John Legend having a date night just over one week after little Luna Simone was born in 2016? People went wild: judging, shaming, and calling her out as a "bad mom" all over the Internet because they left their newborn so soon for a date night. I'm not sure most of us would try to pull that off, but I also think this blissful couple was onto something smart.

Now that my daughters are out of the baby stage (and I have 20/20 hindsight, just as you will when you're out of the baby stage in a few years), I see John and Chrissy's stunt as being a practical symbol for relationships through new parenting: newborns sleep most of the time and the kid was, most likely, very well taken care of during their two-hour absence—so why not celebrate a new family as man and wife if you feel well and it doesn't put your baby at risk? They were famous for their PDA and all-around affection with each other before baby, and that date night seemed to announce, "Yeah, we're still that same couple." Don't fall into a trap of letting an eight-pound bundle of joy change your priorities where your relationship is concerned. Just like John and Chrissy (and Giuliana and Bill), remember that you and your spouse were here first and are a team.

Once you feel like your better half and you are swinging in the same direction (or from the chandelier, ha!), it's time to address your new life—and new love—on a practical level. I'm not talking about shaving legs here; I'm talking about day-to-day duties like diapers, dishes, and doing the laundry. I know there are plenty of men out there who pony up for household duties, but let's face it, many don't.

As an American Armenian who was raised with a dad who didn't quite ever learn the concept of kitchen cleanup (not his fault; it was the way the world worked back then), I was raised in a house where the woman did everything domestically related, whether she had a career or not. Marrying a traditionally raised, American Armenian guy, I planned to run my own household that way, too (it pretty much does run this way to this day, with a few deviations here and there). Hey, as a mover-and-shaker and all-out hustler in the I-can-handle-it-all-kids-work-home-husband-whatever department, I could do it all, every single day, no problem. That got really exhausting really fast. Thank goodness for the unsolicited advice of my older and wiser colleague and friend, Rick Bentley.

Just before I had my first daughter in summer of 2010, I went to a movie screening for press and unexpectedly ran into Rick, the entertainment writer from the *Fresno Bee* newspaper (shout to my hometown of Fresno, California). Rick had always been so kind to me—every time I'd get a new job on television, he'd write an article about it and tell readers to watch and support a local girl taking a crack at her dreams. He's several years older than I and had a son in his early twenties at the time I ran into him here. My belly was ready to pop, and we sat together to watch the film. We caught up on all the usual things you catch up on when someone is pregnant: how work had slowed down since my pregnancy, how kids grow so fast, how I should enjoy every second. . . . Rick also, unexpectedly, dropped one of the most valuable pieces of wisdom that I often suggest to new moms today.

He said, "When the baby's born, figure out one thing that your husband can do right away . . . just one task, one job, something that he's game to do every day as your kid grows. It's the best bonding experience for a dad and it'll give you a break." He continued about how, as a young dad, he opted for bathtime duties. I listened, totally second-guessed him (as I don't ever remember my dad chipping in with manual labor concerning us kids), and then basically forgot about Rick's advice.

But when my daughter was born, things changed: I suddenly discovered how petrified I was to give her a bath! *She's so tiny! I'm going to hurt her! Help me!* Standing over the portable baby bath on top of our kitchen counter, Rick's words shot to the front of my brain.

"Will you bathe her?" I begged my husband (the pediatric surgeon who is used to dealing with squirmy, fragile, screaming small people). "Please? She's so tiny and I'm scared . . ." I'm not one to pull the wimpy, prissy I-can't-do-it card, but this was a chance to get my ducks in a row, an opportunity to cash in and set the standard of practice in my home. *That's it, play scared Jill.* My husband bathed our girl that first time, and the pattern continued for the first few years of both our daughters' lives. Andre soon became a frequent bath-giver at our house. Granted, I gave plenty of baths (still do), but tasking my husband with bathtime sneakily broke the seal to get him involved in some kind of domesticated duty early on.

Does my man do laundry? Hell no, not ever. Does he load the dishwasher? Not unless I beg and complain and throw some kind of cranky-wife fit. Does he bathe the girls when I ask him (so I can clean up the kitchen or just have a few minutes to decompress a bit at the end of the day)? Yes. Does he draw and color with our daughters, take them on outings to Orchard Supply Hardware, and handle the bedtime routine on Thursday nights by himself when I must go to bed early for my 4 a.m. wake up to appear on Friday's early morning news? Yes. I fully credit baby bath-duty for creating this lifestyle. Get the dad in your life involved in one task from the get-go—it will set up a more organized family home life for you in the long run.

3 Fixes for Getting Your Spouse to Help Early On

From Doyin Richards, fatherhood author, public speaker, and founder of DaddyDoinWork.com

The first time I met Doyin, it was at a blogger event celebrating digital legend Jill Smokler of Scary Mommy back in 2013—he was the only guy in the room talking to a bunch of women about sex after babies. He had us hollering with laughter and delightful embarrassment. Doyin also happens to be one of America's most popular "digital dads" changing the expectations and actions of fathers everywhere. He's also the dude who helped spearhead this book. I'm proud to call him my friend. Here's his advice.

1. **Let Dad do things his way**. Nothing turns off dads more than moms who micromanage how they do their jobs as parents. The way your spouse does things may not be your way, or even the right way, but it's *his* way. As long as his child isn't hurt or in danger, let the man do his thing. He'll be much more engaged as a parenting partner that way.

2. **Encourage Dad to spend time with baby** on his own. Let him bond with his baby without Mom around; by taking the baby on a walk, giving the baby a bath, picking out baby's clothes, and even wearing the baby. Simple acts like that will lay the foundation for a daddy-baby bond to last for the rest of their lives.

3. **Don't accept excuses for why he can't be involved.** He worked a long day, he's tired, he doesn't know how to do hair . . . it's all nonsense. Insist that he step up and be the kind of great dad that millions of men are across America. This isn't the 1950s anymore; modern dads read bedtime stories, sing lullabies, and wake up in the middle of the night to change poopy diapers. Don't settle for anything less from your man.

A baby brings dramatic shifts for any couple, no matter how long you've been together. New responsibilities, new stresses, new worries, and a new little person who requires constant attention can be overwhelming at first, but keep forging on because raising a baby together requires love for each other, even if that love seems oddly unfamiliar sometimes. Every single one of my friends have complained and commiserated about the what-the's and why's of this phenomenon over texts, phone calls, and in person. It happens to all of us at different times.

Be aware of what you feel toward your spouse postbaby and commit to staying resilient and actively connected to your partner throughout your journey as new parents. If and when you find yourself feeling like something has jumped a track or is missing a link in your relationship, don't panic or waste time—do what works for your relationship to readjust your love for each other so you can revel in the joy of being parents. A happy heart is imperative to keeping a bounceback active.

Want to know what else is imperative? Being loud. Being very, very loud . . .

Loud Love with Your Baby.

One of the things that send many new moms into emotional tailspins during the first few months is the physical and emotional isolation that can come at home with a newborn. You know, the whole OMG-I'm-stuck-at-home-alone-in-a-Groundhog-Day-state-with-no-one-to-talk-to realization. Most of us live far away from family and don't typically go outside to hang out with neighbors on the front porch. (If you have family close by, or if you regularly hang out with your neighbors, I envy you!)

Some of us feel the newborn isolation more than others, like one of my friends who can't stand staying home at all costs, while some of us actually enjoy it. Where's the village? Where's the social comfort? Where's the noise? The self-awareness of extreme isolation, I've found, usually happens leading up to the thirty-day mark. A productive bounce-back depends on conquering this time period.

But Jill! Didn't you say that the first thirty days are lockdown mode and that you should focus on the "job" of finding your rhythm as a mother with a new baby? Yes, I did say that. Thank you for listening! Staying at home in those early days, in your underwear (just like we talked about), is vital to discovering your own pace and cadence for tending to baby and yourself those early months. It's challenging but necessary work that might seem mind-numbing after you've been functioning on broken sleep for a few weeks—especially if you're an extremely social person or worked in a fast-paced career before baby. Being at home might make you loopy because you suddenly find yourself in quiet solitude (minus a baby's noises, of course). The solution? Create your own social scene at home and start talking aloud.

Talk to yourself? No! Talk to your baby. Even though there were two of us at home, I still remember how empty my apartment felt when my husband was at work in those early, first-time-mom weeks. I had visitors pop in here and there, but most of my friends worked, so no one was coming over to hang out with me day in and day out. The loneliness of being a brand-new mother blindsided me—I was the girl who always preferred to go shopping by myself, found comfort taking in an afternoon movie alone, and even savored having lunch totally solo before the days of smart phone companionship. But now, with a newborn, I felt a bit lost. I wasn't working at the time, and man, did I miss the fast-paced vigor of my job! (Remember, I *talk* for a living.)

I overcompensated for my loneliness using every trick in the book; I played music, I flipped on the television, I called friends on the phone or emailed my former colleagues between baby duties and during her naps. And then, I realized, I wasn't alone at home . . . I had a *baby*! Why not start talking aloud to the person I was spending all my days with?

My daughter was my new partner in crime, mascot, best friend, and all-around motivator to get life together. So I started talking to her in ways that I'd talk to my husband, friends, or past roommates. "Good morning! How are you? Isn't it a beautiful day? Although, I am really tired today. . . . What was that last night—you didn't want to sleep? I was thinking, if you're in the mood later, maybe we should try some tummy time? Or maybe you can chill in your yellow rocking chair while I get myself a bagel? Is that okay? Do you want a bagel? I know, you don't have teeth yet . . . but you will soon, cutie-pie! Damn! I'm out of cream cheese. Let's see if I have any jam. You're going to like jam when you get older; it tastes just like candy."

On and on I'd continue, talking to my little one as though she were going to sit up at the age of three weeks and tell me she didn't like cream cheese. Yes, she'd cry as any newborn cries, but I'd continue talking to her as I filled her needs. "I know . . . I agree . . . I am slow at getting this bottle together right now, huh? Hang in there, it's coming honey. What? You're not hungry? Do you have a dirty diaper? Oh my, I'm a silly mommy—your diaper is dirty and I didn't even notice! Am I fired? Let's go change you. . . . Come on, get a move on."

I'd lay her on the bed and ask her about her day. I'd plop her in her chair and make comments about how I should really do a load of laundry before Daddy comes home. I'd position her on my knees, facing me, as I sat on our couch with my feet propped up on my coffee table and question her about whether she liked her bottle. She'd just stare at me, eyes wide open, soaking everything in. I also used my teeny tiny captive audience to revisit my musical theater days of singing and performing from high school and college. (I'd try to hit those high notes like I did when I was twenty-one years old—no, the pipes didn't work like they used to, folks, but it didn't matter.) We'd read all kind of books, because most every television host needs to keep their cold reading teleprompter chops up should there suddenly be an audition to replace the host of *Access Hollywood* or something.

Why so chatty? It was the only tactic that kept me from feeling absolutely alone. I stayed away from baby talk (well, maybe I did just a little for those days my girls looked extra squishy and precious) and just opted for regular conversation as though she were a real person. *Babies are real people, right?*

Talking brought me back to life—I soon started feeling like my world was spinning and rockin' and rollin'. When my second daughter was born a year and a half later, I did the same thing out of not knowing what else to do. Our household conversations kept me alive, communicating, and happy (by this time my older child was fully talking, too—I credit our long conversations together when she was a baby). Sure, I could've enrolled us in a newborn mommy group (as many of my friends did), but I just wasn't interested in it at the time. I didn't want to sign up for the hassle of having to be somewhere on a certain day, at a certain time. Staying home and focusing on "learning my baby" was adding up to work in a most positive way for me in the long run.

Turns out, I was unknowingly setting up my newborns for early developmental success by talking, singing, and reading throughout our days. Babies crave conversation on a most scientifically proven level. Did you know that more than 80 percent of a child's brain is developed by their third birthday? (I didn't when I was doing all this talking and performing for my infant.) According to research, newborns can immediately recognize their mom's voice; the more we talk to them, the more secure our babies feel. (And the less they cry, perhaps?)

Studies also prove that language skills and vocabulary start developing from the day children are born—so tell your caregivers to talk, and talk often! According to the early childhood organization First 5 California (here in my home state), talking, reading, and singing to a child from birth is the best way to boost psychological and social development that also establishes a stronger love for learning later on. Had I known all this during my days as a new mom, I would've thought myself a wicked genius, rather than the crazy lady talking to her baby in the corner apartment.

But how to combat a baby's crying . . . and crying . . . and crying? I can't speak to dealing with colic (my second daughter was notoriously fussy and loud and screaming most of the time, although not clinically colicky), but I can offer how I interpreted her crying in a way that helped me on a personal level: I reminded myself she was *talking* to me. Every time she cried, I took deep breaths to calm myself down (because it drove me nuts) and kept telling myself to interpret her noise as a signal for what she was trying to tell me and how I could fix it. (This goes back to being a resilient, problem-solving CEO of all things baby.)

As she'd cry, I'd talk back to her. "Is your diaper wet?" Nope. "Are you hungry?" Nope. "Are you tired? Are you swaddled tight enough?" Nope. Crying is a prompt for a parent to solve the situation at hand—that's it. A good friend of mine once told me that crying is just a baby talking to you, and that helped me cope on many days.

I'm always one to panic first, but committing to staying calm and turning the crying into a "game" that motivated me to solve the mystery of what the heck the issue was kept me semi-sane (most of the time). Some days you will score, some days you won't score. Accept the randomness of it all *(no fails here!)* and move on, moment by moment. Just because you might not figure it out one day doesn't mean you won't figure it out the next day. Talking is therapeutic by nature, and its effects add up in the most positive ways—so talk, for yourself and your baby. Now that you know the power of loud love, you've got to get tough. . . .

Tough Love with Yourself.

Parenting isn't for the weak, so you've got to suck it up, sister. A bounceback requires that a new mom act like a boss no matter what (there's that CEO thing again). While seasoned mothers and postpartum experts usually advise rookie moms to go extra easy on our choices, I'm going to suggest we do the opposite in a most vigilant way; the first few months is the time to get tough about making choices. Without even considering babies, we women are stereotypically and shamefully insistent about questioning our own actions, deciding on something, doubting it all again, and then sometimes weeping because we're so freaking tired of questioning everything so much.

According to a bit of research led by Dove in early 2016 (yes, the beauty company), four out of five negative comments about women online came from . . . wait for it . . . ourselves! (Yes, women. Pathetic.) If we're so good at tearing ourselves down and doubting ourselves, then we surely have the grit to shift our thinking to make ourselves feel self-assured on a day-to-day basis. A new mom must get tough about filling up our own confidence tanks regularly, for the good of our long-term parenting skills and stamina. Confidence grows when committed effort is involved.

How to start filling up that tank? Schedule time with yourself in the mirror (hey, if you're mostly going to be on some kind of home lockdown for six weeks or more with a newborn anyway, might as well fill the time in a way that's going to be positively productive). During these thirty days of newborn life, try setting a timer or alarm to ring three times throughout the day (without waking baby, of course). When it rings, march your sweet, underwear-clad self over to the nearest mirror, look at your reflection, and say something nice to your own face. There's nothing to be embarrassed about—no one except your baby will hear you, and I'll bet he won't tell anyone.

At the risk of sounding like a hippy-dippy zenbot, consider this: positive affirmations done regularly are widely credited to reverse and purge negative thoughts, which then lead to a more fulfilled and productive life. What to say to your reflection? I'll give you three go-to phrases that worked for me; these originated from a fabulous man by the name of John Hall, my theater coach at UCLA, when he was teaching a class full of music nerds (myself included) how to be successful performers on stage almost twenty years ago. His words were so wise back then, they've stuck with me all the way through motherhood, and I found myself saying these to my reflection in my new mom days. I continue to say them now:

- ☺ *Tits up!* (Good posture and perky boobs make anyone feel better instantly.)
- ☺ *Bigger idiots than me have figured this out.* (So I will, too, because I'm smarter than those other idiots.)
- ☺ *Even if I feel like I'm doing it wrong, I will be strong.* (Strong always wins . . . because strong is confident no matter what.)

Maybe John should've also taught a class for new parents. Making an effort to offer your best, even on a day that might feel like your worst day ever, is all you can do. Find satisfaction in giving whatever effort you can handle on any given day and then move on and forget about it. If your voice feels raspy, just sing the best you can and be done. If your baby refuses to take a nap and you're at a loss for trying to get her down, just do your best and don't hem and haw about why it's not working. Tomorrow is another performance. Tomorrow is another effort. Tomorrow will most likely be better. If it's not? There will be a day after that. Keep your tits up—babies have a thing for boobs, remember?

What's the catch for making these phrases effective? You must believe what you say. Get bossy about giving your reflection compliments and then give yourself permission to believe them throughout the day. If you don't say them when motherhood is fresh, you might not ever hear them as much as you truly need to. (That baby can't talk yet, remember?) You're responsible for filling your confidence tank in a tough-talking way, because infants usually react more favorably to confident mothers. Babies are like little animals; they can smell fear and take you out in a split second.

Know what else can us out in a split second? Doubt about our own first-time skills. Don't be afraid to treat your first child as though you've already had another baby before. It takes steep imagination and calculated delusion, but pretending you've already done this new mom thing will season the way you approach some of motherhood's most nerve-inducing deeds.

Talk to any second-, third-, or fourth-time mom about how she treated her first child compared with the babies she had afterward. I guarantee she'll laugh about how uptight she acted. She'll also probably share how relaxed she was about not rinsing pacifiers, using unsterilized bottles, and letting her second, third, or fourth babies cry in their cribs for thirty more seconds in the morning so she could brush her teeth and pee before launching into mom-mode. I myself am now confused about why I always felt like I didn't have time to bathe with only one immobile baby in my house—and why I felt the need to bring my newborn's rolling bassinet into the bathroom while I showered, just so I could watch her, while she was perfectly safe! Most new mama drama associated with our firstborns *(we must sterilize! we must wash everything! we must not shower in the name of not ever taking our eyes off the baby!)* is caused by us, and not our babies.

The quicker you realize that babies really don't supply more upheaval than adults create or feed into (aside from the needing to eat and sleep every few hours), and the sooner you realize that babies aren't *that* complicated, the easier new life with baby will be. I'm not suggesting you won't have drama (can I tell you about those times my youngest daughter projectile vomited all over my white couches with a roomful of family and friends?), but don't waste valuable time making your life a high-maintenance, nervous wreck if there's no cause for it. We're in charge of how much drama a baby brings, not the other way around.

For me, getting tough meant not bothering to sterilize bottles and not freaking out that I hadn't vacuumed the carpet in a few days should I need to lay my daughter on it to change her diaper. Most times, I didn't rinse that pacifier, either (five-second rule, you know). And, sometimes, I let my babies sit and play on the lawn with only diapers on . . . and sometimes they'd even eat bits of dirt! (This coming from a woman who is seriously petrified of snails, worms, and those creepy roly-poly bugs that hang out between blades of grass.) But I listened to stories and wisdom from moms before me and decided I'd also done this baby thing before *in my head* and it all turned out fine the first time. You've got this, too.

How else did I keep my heart in the right place so that my mind and body could follow? I made the toughest call of all according to what my heart kept telling me: I opted to be a mostly stay-at-home mom for the first year of both my daughters' lives. (Consider this my most unexpected advice in this "tough calls" portion of the program.) Granted, I was launching my blog and pursuing random television side jobs to keep one foot in the career game over baby's first years, but I was able to financially opt out of working full time, and, man, did it make a difference in the long run for me.

Even though I started this bounce back experiment to return to working on television after babies, I couldn't bear the thought of leaving my newborn babies with caretakers so I could maintain demands of what my full-time career entailed (weekdays, plus some nights and weekends). Leaving a two- or three-month-old baby in the hands of a background-checked stranger from 8 a.m. to 7 p.m. every day, five days a week, can be tough for any new mom. I'd have felt flat-out jealous if a stranger got to spend more time with my baby than I did that first year.

Yes, a lot of women are obligated to do it and get used to it, but I decided to take my career to idling mode, keeping one foot in, during the baby years. We could afford our mortgage and moderate life expenses without me working full time, so that's how we rolled. Yes, I was lucky and I am thankful. Taking myself out of the full-speed, full-time career game pissed off my ambition a bit but made the rest of me feel content.

My friend and Los Angeles news reporter Stephanie Stanton fessed up to me how doing the same thing made her happier as a new mom. After her second (and last) baby was born, she took the pressure off herself to return to work immediately. "I decided to savor every moment with my new baby daughter. To me, being FAB means having the confidence to know that work will always be there . . . but precious newborn moments are fleeting."

Want some celebrity backup? Actresses Eva Mendes, Mila Kunis, Jennifer Garner, and Jessica Biel have all talked about taking their careers down a notch after becoming mothers—a few of them also allegedly opting out of having nannies, too. (All this written at the risk that you mistake Stephanie and me for entitled or lazy women.

I beg you not to think that, because we are career-minded, hard-working people who happened to make a choice that was available to us, felt right at the time, and was equally unexpected for us, too!)

Being a mostly stay-at-home mom during the first year also freed me from that "working new mom doubt and guilt" you might hear about, which was huge. *I feel so bad I'm not there at home with him. . . . When I'm at work, my mind is on what's at home and when I'm at home, my mind is on what's at work. . . .* You know, *that.* Did I have a twinge of guilt or feel bummed when I missed my daughter's very first steps because I traveled to New York to audition for that job at HLN? Nope, I didn't. I'd been home with my sweet girl for an entire year, working random freelance jobs in between, and saw most all the other firsts and everys up until then.

Because I was home more than I wasn't those first several months, my daughter and I established a rock-solid bond, free of the dramatic push-pull that many new moms feel if they return to work full speed weeks after baby is born. She may've taken her first steps, but I didn't have that hankering, guilty feeling that I missed something because I'd been there throughout everything else. Does that make sense? I had been with her more than I hadn't been with her, so I felt more ready when I did return to work more frequently later.

Did I have days when I cursed my at-home status and wanted to tear my hair out for changing my shirt *again* because I just got spit up on *again*? Yes! I missed my fast-paced career like all women who love their careers inevitably do when they take a step back! However, I found personal peace doing what I felt the right thing was for my own set of values and situation in the long run, which meant clocking in quality time with baby early on and shifting my career into idling mode (still running, but not really going anywhere).

All of this spilled, being a full-time working mom during baby's first year isn't a negative thing! I have plenty of friends who couldn't wait to get back to work and slipped into full-time working mom mode easily. I admire them! New moms *can and should* work if they want or need to, but I'm just calling attention to being honest about your own emotions and the options available to you per your economic situation. Whatever choice your spirit is pulling you toward, own it regardless of what anyone else might think. If you want to return to work at full speed, then do it! *You do you.* But expect that it will be a juggle and hustle in different ways.

Samantha Ettus, work-life balance expert and author—and personal role model of mine when it comes to fostering a fulfilling life and career while raising a family—kept me treading steadily through the early years of motherhood with some most frank advice. When I started working more this last year, and started questioning whether I was trying to juggle too much with family and career, she told me: "It is easy to blame work for anything that goes wrong in your personal life. Don't! Things go wrong whether you are working or not. Maintaining your career will keep you happier and more fulfilled in the long run . . . this includes working during the sleepless new mom years." It's not easy to keep balls in the air with a new baby, but you can't really bounce if you don't have balls. (Gotcha!)

Don't apologize for your feelings, whatever way they may swing, and be practical about circumstances you might need to maintain for economic purposes of supporting your family. Eight of out of ten moms work, and 40 percent of moms who work are the family's primary breadwinner. If you do need to return to your career but are feeling unsettled about going into the office five days a week, think about investigating flex-work options with your employer.

Do you remember that dramatic new parental leave policy that Netflix implemented a few years ago—that salaried and a designated group of hourly employees could take paid parental leave for up to a full year after a child's birth or adoption? (Compare that to US law only requiring companies to offer twelve weeks of maternity leave to eligible new mothers.) More and more companies have been following suit, and the push for increased parental leave (including leave for dads) is on the rise.

Flex-work opportunities vary across state lines, but once you start educating yourself about little-known loopholes or undercover options that might exist, your maternity leave might get to be longer than you first thought. Many of my friends who work at companies (non-entertainment related) have been allowed to do their jobs from home a few days a week over the first year of baby's life. I have some friends who work full-time hours at home and some who are only obligated to go into the office two or three days a week. Start talking and asking questions to like-minded women who've been there, whom you can trust at your company, to make your work *work* for you.

3 Fixes for Creating a Longer Maternity Leave

From Allyson Downey, founder of weeSpring.com & author of Here's the Plan: Your Practical, Tactical Guide to Advancing Your Career During Pregnancy and Parenthood

I first met Ally when she launched her wildly successful baby gear referral site weeSpring.com in 2012; she was sharp and focused on serving new parents in a most resourceful way. I was fascinated by how she seemed to forge ahead effortlessly in her career with babies at home at the same time! Here are some of Ally's most insightful quick tips for how to navigate maternity leave and beyond (be sure to check out her book for details; this is only the tip of the iceberg):

1. **Don't shy away from negotiating.** While 57 percent of men are ready to negotiate in the workplace, only 7 percent of women do. We're taught from an early age to be gracious and grateful, so the idea of asking for more than what's offered feels uncomfortable. Push through that discomfort by reminding yourself that you're asking for what you're worth—and you're worth a *lot*. The cost of replacing you is considerable.

2. **Get creative.** I prep for every negotiation by brainstorming a thorough list of what's on the table. For maternity leave, it could include when you return, the hours that you work, where you're working, and all combinations therein, such as working from home three days a week or working part-time for three months after maternity leave. I also advise women to talk in three-month increments; you can always ask to extend an arrangement, and something that feels "temporary" and makes it a lot easier for your manager to accept. Be bold in what you're asking for; as noted above, a guy in your shoes would be.

3. **Frame everything for what's in it for them.** A major "don't" is leading with a sentence like, "I'd like more time off to bond with my baby." Don't get me wrong, that's a great reason. But think about the advantages to your

> company and speak in those terms. "Working remotely two days a week will reduce my commuting time, so I can get an hour back in my schedule on those days to get ahead on XYZ projects," or "I'll be available for some calls and emails in my fourth month of parental leave, and then I'll be able to jump back in 100 percent in December."

Another tough call I made was opting out of hiring consistent help because I had a new baby. That's right, no nanny (minus trusted and referred sitters who came and went when I scored random freelance jobs here and there). While most new moms don't ever think about getting a full-time nanny to help with baby, finding a nanny or night nurse in Los Angeles is almost an assumed norm when a baby is born whether you're a working mom or stay-at-home mom. (It's a bit ridiculous, honestly.)

Here's the reality: if you return to work after baby, you're going to need a caretaker for obvious and practical reasons. But if you're planning to be home with baby, day in and day out, then I'd argue it best serves you to hunker down, do the manual labor, and build an uninterrupted and solid foundation for getting to know your child during the newborn days and beyond—minus the breaks you take to get out of the house by yourself once in a while (we all need those to refresh).

In the words of a very, very wealthy friend of mine—someone who's done a fantastic job raising nice, unentitled kids in an over-the-top material world and who also opted out of getting any kind of nanny for her three kids: "The more help you get, the more help you need." It's true. Running a marathon is exponentially more

159

challenging and downright dangerous if you don't interval train for it first. Hitting the high notes in a song won't happen if you don't commit to doing your vocal exercises and rehearsing every day. Passing that exam isn't going to happen if you don't study for it consistently. Everything you do with baby—feeding, swaddling, rocking, burping, diaper changing—contributes to making each future day as a parent a bit easier for you, because you're putting your time in to train, gain experience, build stamina, and earn depth of wisdom that you will count on to shape your parenting decisions and abilities as baby grows.

But it's just so hard. I need someone to come in here and help me out. I agree! If you find yourself buried, then get practical relief as you need it. Once a week? Twice a week? A lady who comes and irons every Saturday morning? Go for it. I'm just suggesting you stop yourself from hiring that full-time help *just because you might be able to afford it.* Here's what I've seen to be true with many smart and capable women: a full-time nanny can sometimes get in the way of a stay-at-home mom's ability to fully figure out her baby's needs and habits. If a nanny is picking up baby from his nap, feeding him, tickling his toes with that fluffy white bunny your cousin sent as a surprise, and taking care of his every need (because she's doing her job well), then where will you stand as the in-home mom of the house?

Relying on help, if you're also home, might just prevent you from gaining valuable problem-solving skills that you need to draw on for future parenting situations. Nannies tend to know what they're doing because they have experience, so opt out of being cheated from collecting your own experience for the big picture. (Nannies everywhere are now calling for my demise.) Taking initiative to hustle baby management when tough times called early on taught me how to problem-solve in ways that benefit me to this day. If I hadn't put the time into problem-solving what worked effectively to get my youngest daughter to nap (man, did she resist), I'd have never figured out what worked and what didn't when it was time to put her to bed at night. Resilience comes when you commit to learning and developing it in reasonable, consistent spurts over time. *The more help you get, the more help you need.*

All this said, if you're really feeling overwhelmed beyond what you think is normal and expected—emotionally or mentally, to the point where you want to run away and never come back—then you must get tough quickly and react to your own needs, ASAP. Postpartum anxiety and depression (known as PPD) are serious and affect approximately one in seven pregnant and new moms by diminishing feelings of self-worth, destroying confidence, and ruining friendships and relationships. These very real conditions are nothing to be ashamed of; they are biochemical circumstances that need expert medical attention to overcome.

Actress Hayden Panettiere sought treatment for PPD twice after the birth of her daughter, talk show host Tamera Mowry-Housely of *The Real* once said she felt a "black cloud" after her son's birth in 2013, and powerhouse Grammy-winning vocalist Adele went on the record in *Vanity Fair* magazine to say how scared she is to have another baby because of the PPD she experienced with her son. If you find yourself feeling helplessly defeated or just "off," talk to your doctor and seek guidance so that you can continue to bounce back in a healthy way, mentally and emotionally.

3 Fixes for Figuring Out if Your Feelings Need Help—Quick

From Katherine Stone, mom, founder & CEO of PostpartumProgress.org

I first discovered Katherine and her cause for educating women about postpartum depression online years ago. I hadn't experienced PPD, but her mission and message deeply affected me (maybe because I'm so passionate about this bouncing back thing). I was thankful to meet her for the first time in early 2016 as I was writing this book; she was warm, friendly, and beyond effervescent about keeping women healthy in every way after birthing babies and beyond. I'm honored to have her wisdom included.

1. **Sleep is everything!** If you can't sleep when the baby is sleeping, and I mean "Oh my god, I'm completely exhausted and still can't fall asleep and why am I staring at the ceiling at 3 a.m. night after night? What is wrong with me?!?!?!" kind of can't sleep, call your doctor. Sometimes the inability to sleep even when you want to is a sign of postpartum depression, or a sign that you might be developing it. Getting support can get you back on track and get you the crucial sleep you need to function. (The same thing is true, by the way, if you find you've completely lost your appetite. Talk to your doc!)

2. **Feelings aren't facts.** For nearly 20 percent of all moms, having a new baby doesn't feel anything like the blissful

experience they thought it would. If after the first couple of weeks postpartum you are feeling lost, anxious, disconnected, miserable, or like you don't recognize yourself anymore, you might be struggling with a very common but also very treatable maternal mental illness like PPD. If your brain tells you that you are a terrible person and have no business being a mother, *it's lying to you*. Call your doctor.

3. **Self-care isn't selfish**. Many moms think that taking time away from baby for exercise, coffee with friends, a support group, or a psychotherapy appointment is selfish. I can't focus on myself, there's no time! Oh yes there is, friend. You didn't check your own humanity at the door when you became a mother. You must take the time to ensure you are as healthy and strong as you can be, both physically and emotionally. You can't help your baby if you haven't helped yourself first.

12 FAST FIXES
TO KEEP YOU FOCUSED THE FIRST FEW MONTHS

Okay, here it is: a simple set of rules I personally invented to push typical new mama drama away and launch organization and routine during the first few months. Following these tips will help keep your focus and resilience thriving.

1. ***Fix your bed before 10 a.m.*** This perky habit should start within the first month of bringing baby home, as doing this task will fire up your spirit to tackle the day no matter how many spit-up waterfalls get hurled at you in a two-hour time frame. Ask any Navy SEAL about this and they will tell you how the mundane act of bed fixing will positively motivate you, as one completed task is usually followed by another completed task (like brushing your teeth), and so on. You don't have to do it perfectly; you just need to do it. Any chance you remember that viral 2014 commencement speech for the University of Texas at Austin from Admiral William

H. McRaven? He sternly told a bunch of new college gradu-
ates heading into the workforce, "And if by chance you have a
miserable day, you come back home to a bed that is made . . .
that you made. And a made bed gives you encouragement that
tomorrow will be better." He's right. How did I get my bed
fixed at my house (most) every day? I laid my newborns in my
sheets, which made pulling up the blankets fun and funny. I'd
giggle and make faces at each of my daughters as I made the
bed around them, and they'd smile back at me. Bed making
was part of our morning playtime. And yes, I did feel better
each and every day my bed was made.

2. *Drink caffeine on a schedule.* Thanks to broken sleep patterns,
you're going to need energy. Coffee, Coke, Pepsi, Mountain
Dew, or Red Bull provide a blasts of vigor, period. Find the
formula that works for you and stick to it. For me, drinking
one cup of coffee in the morning and one glass of soda right
after lunch (sometimes a splash more here and there, if I needed
it) kept me functioning until bedtime. Since I opted out of
nursing, I had zero concern about caffeine entering the baby's
bloodstream via breast milk. (Aha!) Many of us abused coffee
before babies (I'm lookin' at you, lady), so what's the difference
after babies? Having a newborn is no time to kick harmless
habits that worked for you before motherhood (as long as those
habits aren't life-threatening).

3. *Drink water on a schedule.* This might seem counterproductive
to the self-induced caffeine trip, but this tip is purely here for
health reasons. When my babies were newborns, I remember
not even thinking about eating or drinking anything simply
because I was running on adrenaline and on a freakish my-new-
baby-is-so-cute high (which you will soon understand). Red

alert: your body needs water—and food—so make sure you give it what it needs. Otherwise, heart palpitations and bouts of insomnia due to dehydration may follow.

4. ***Don't bother heating formula/milk (for bottle-feeding).*** My mom was always shocked about how I never heated up my daughters' formula to feed them. It's not like I was giving them freezing-cold bottles, I was just giving them room temperature milk! The truth is, heating up bottles is an extra step that you can afford to skip in order to have more time for something else. (To lie down? To put away that laundry?) A baby gets accustomed to whatever you start doing and will most likely not recoil at room-temperature formula as long as you're consistent with giving it to them. Some moms say their babies experienced stomach issues (gas, etc.) when they served bottles that were not warmed up. I never heated anything up from Day One, and my girls drank like normal babies and developed perfectly fine. Not to mention, I like to think this also taught them to be low-maintenance for taking bottles. Don't start a habit you can't follow through on (perfectly warmed bottles). Don't waste time doing things that don't matter in the long run. Minutes add up, and new moms need as many extra minutes as we can get.

5. ***Skip the sterilization.*** Those snazzy sanitizing tubs that you load your bottles into and pop into the microwave (after you wash them) to make sure each and every germ is eradicated simply aren't necessary. You might think you need one to "be safe" so that your child doesn't contract a strange virus that could've been kept away, but you don't. I bought one of those sterilization tubs but then stopped short of using it when my husband laughed at my using it and said, "Those things don't

sterilize. The second you touch that bottle again it's back to square one. Hot water and mild soap work perfectly well to keep things clean." I'm not one to question a surgeon with twelve-plus years of intensive training and experience involving true practices of sterilization . . . so . . . I quickly stopped wasting time sterilizing my feeding tools that weren't really getting sterilized anyway.

6. *Hang a mirror in your kitchen.* Not only does seeing your reflection in the main area of your home make you more likely to say those tough-talking, positive affirmations to yourself throughout the day, but it also encourages a speedy return to applying makeup. Here's the tip I tell every new mom friend who can't seem to understand how or why I managed to smear on concealer, mascara, blush, and lip gloss most mornings when I had a sixteen-month-old and a newborn under my roof at one time: stash some minimal makeup into one of your kitchen drawers for superfast access and application in the kitchen. The more mirrors you have accessible, the more likely you'll use them. And, oh yeah, any makeup should be quickly applied sometime before noon.

7. *Get offline.* This unexpected advice coming from a woman who launched a blog and joined every single social media channel available when her babies were newborns so that I could work in the digital space . . . and who is still online in a most involved and questionably self-centered way? Yes. Here's what I really mean when I say get offline: don't get carried away clicking on every article you scan that details "the hidden health meanings of how often your baby spits up, cries, poops, or sleeps during the day" should you be concerned about how often your baby spits up, cries, poops, or sleeps during the

day. Get my drift? The Internet is an awesome place to guide us toward solutions and decipher benign mysteries that our babies present us with, but don't get obsessed about reading often-uniformed and incorrect info. The Internet can scare the crap out of you if you open yourself up to it. If you're truly concerned about something pertaining to you or your baby, take it offline (out of Facebook mommy groups!) and head to your doctor to address the issue. Additionally, getting offline as much as you can will keep your brain functioning in a more calm and controlled way. It's been proven that the brain reacts to too much online stimulation in a similar way as it would if it were high on cocaine. Don't be a mom on drugs.

8. ***Empty the kitchen sink every night.*** This was always a nonnegotiable for me unless I was ill or seriously pissed off and trying to make a point about household duties with my husband or something. (Who am I kidding, this tip is *still* is a nonnegotiable with me.) An empty sink before you go to bed, whether the dishwasher is full of dirty or clean dishes, will make you feel better when you wake up and head into your kitchen the next day. Starting your morning with a stinky sink full of plates is no way to begin a new day. (This is the other end of the making-the-bed spectrum, I guess.)

9. ***Preset your overnight feeding requirements on your nightstand.*** The power to avoid bumping into furniture in the dark while making your way into the kitchen to find a bottle as your baby screams for dear hunger in the middle of the night lies with you. Get organized for those overnight feedings before hitting the sack: set up your nightstand with premeasured formula (in plastic baggies or compartmentalized snack containers) and prefilled bottles of perfectly measured water so that all you have

to do is be half-awake to dump the powder into the already-filled bottle, screw on the nipple, give it a good shake, and feed baby in one swift movement. For the first few months, I'd set up three to four premeasured bottles, which slowly diminished to one to two bottles as baby eventually learned to sleep longer between feedings (you'll see how this progresses as your baby grows). This minimizes the need for you to be totally conscious while giving a bottle in those wee hours. (Your spouse will also appreciate this organization, since he might be giving a bottle overnight, too.)

10. *Attempt outings after you feed baby at home.* I'm notorious for taking my girls everywhere from the market to the mall in the very early months of their lives (after our thirty-day lockdown, that is), yet I could never relate to many of my friends' tales about how taking babies in public was so difficult to handle. Every time I opted to take the babies out, I'd feed them at home, comfortably, first. Nobody got in the car until my ladies' bellies were full and satisfied. I'd also sometimes load them up when I knew they'd be tired and ready for a nap, so I'd get to drive with a dozing (i.e., not crying) baby in the backseat. What happens if you need to head to an appointment but it's not quite time to feed baby yet? Give them a top-off of milk just before the trip anyway, just for insurance. Saving yourself extra trouble midtrip is most always worth it, even if it does bend the rules of your eat/sleep/play schedule a bit.

11. *No $hit Talk.* Meaning, absolutely no conversations with friends about baby poop, diapers, crap, pee-pee, gaseousness, and/or farting of any kind. I challenge you to resist the urge to loudly announce, "Fire down below!" should your dainty babe have a movement in the presence of visitors. Yeah, it might be funny to announce your baby's bowel movements (most all parents

think so, you'll see), but avoiding $hit-talk is bigger than the obvious yuck factor. Avoiding $hit-talk in the early days of baby makes a stoic promise to yourself, your spouse, your family, and your friends that you will miraculously hold on to a shred of prebaby manners and priorities through this new parenthood thing. Friends who don't have kids yet don't want to hear about your new baby's potty patterns, and friends who do have kids will marvel at your impressive ability to resist having conversations about whether your baby's poop is mustard yellow or dark brown. It's the truth. (You'll soon see how all-consuming the poop-talk can get when a newborn enters the picture.)

12. ***Keep the diaper bag loaded.*** Water bottle? Check. Five diapers? Check. Premeasured formula? Check. Extra socks and onesies? Check. Burp cloth and blanket? Plastic bags (for wet/dirty clothes)? Check. Check. That favorite power bar with all the chocolate chips and cherry chunks in it when you're starving? Check. If you keep your diaper bag packed with supplies and ready to go at all times, you cut your getting-ready prep in half when it's time to actually leave the house with baby. And remember: you don't need to pack the whole nursery! Who says leaving the house with a newborn is hard? Get down with your FAB self.

The most important tip to remember while following these rules? Stay mindful about them while you do them. Focusing on each task that you undertake, *as you do it,* is credited for developing resilience and promoting satisfaction in everyday life. (Aha!) Don't fantasize about where you wish you could go to lunch as you fix your bed. Opt out of mentally checking off the to-do list for tomorrow as you line up those prefilled bottles on your nightstand. Concentrate on one thing at a time, task by task, as you go through your daily motions. Actors call this technique "staying present," organizational experts call this being mindful, I call it survival and success secrets of the most resilient new mothers.

FAB tip! On getting dressed . . .

Even though we talked about hanging around in your most fun undies all day for the first few weeks, you do want to make a point of getting dressed. (This was one of the first tips Ali Landry sent me when I asked her about offering insight for this book.) "Even though you want to stay in your nursing bra and stained nightgown day and night for days in a row it is important for you to just put on something that makes you feel good about yourself," she wrote. And, she's right. Mark your calendar to get a bit dressed up every Friday, if you must. Seeing yourself look like the stylish you before baby does some powerful things for the mind and spirit. Does this explain that time I threw on a brand new, lacy Free People blouse just to clean my own toilets when my firstborn was a few months old? Maybe. And man, did I feel like a million bucks that day.

PART 4
CONQUERING
THE BABY MONTHS
(Month 4 through First Year)

"My biggest fear about becoming a mom would have to be that I am actually good at it. I worry that, no matter how much I read or try to learn before the baby gets here, I won't be prepared enough to be really good at it. But I guess that's a common fear. . . ."
—Debbie Matenopoulos, mom, television host, and bestselling author (June 2014)

Welcome to the fun part, mama. By now, baby's most likely laughed, can hold her head up, is on some kind of organized feed/wake/sleep schedule, and you've maybe even pranced around in some of your prebaby clothes. Now that you're coming out of the delicious and delirious newborn haze, you're in for some major entertainment: plopping up your babe like a stuffed animal, watching him scoot and crawl and smooch solid messy foods all over everything. You're soon in for more chunky-sweet baby glee that you can handle. I remember hitting the four-month mark with both my babes, and it felt pretty damn good. You're back to feeling in sync with yourself and are hopefully feeling in sync with your bundle, too. But look out now! The fourth month is also a most telling test for how committed you truly are to a real bounceback. Once again, we'll start with the brain. . . .

CHAPTER 7
YOUR BABY BRAIN

E ver heard of Mommy Brain? You know, forgetting some thing someone literally just told you five seconds ago because you're so tired or distracted? We all live with Mommy Brain (or, as some call it, Baby Brain). You know, that notion of being a hot mess, feeling defeated, and outright exhausted at the thought of trying to get something done? (Admittedly I still have my moments, too. It's an ongoing and unavoidable by-product of motherhood.) But it is possible to keep Mommy Brain in control and steer yourself to being resilient when it comes to thinking "I can't" or "I shouldn't." Since you might already have a nice case of Mommy Brain (or, Pregnancy Brain), let's remind ourselves of the short list I shared at the start of this guide about how to foster resilience:

- *Facing things that scare you.* (Tackle your fears!)
- *Developing an ethical code to guide daily decisions.* (Organize your day!)
- *Building a strong network of social support.* (Find fun friends!)
- *Making physical exercise a habit.* (Work your body? Better your brain!)
- *Develop mindfulness.* (Learn to stay in the moment and concentrate on *what* you're doing *when* you're doing it.)

Remember these tips? Feel free to memorize them again if you've forgotten. They will help combat any and all Baby Brain, Mommy Brain, and Where-Is-My-Brain feelings that sneak up on us as new mothers. Bouncing back hinges on keeping everything in check while problem solving, including what you attempt do with a baby in tow. Let's start with some simple decisions.

Pee? Yes. Pedicure? Absolutely.

Before you discard this section as a pathetic excuse to include bathroom humor about how a woman's bladder changes after pregnancy, think again, my fabulous friend. The peeing in this section tells a true story about our own problem-solving potential as mothers. The way we think of ourselves is often shaped by what we think we're capable of doing. Successful problem solving *and doing* with your baby in tow will sharpen your confidence and flex your resilience muscles. For me, peeing with my baby on my lap proved everything I ever needed to know about myself as a new mom.

When my first daughter was about seven months old, I was driving us back home to Los Angeles from a mommy-and-me weekend visit at my parents' house in Fresno, California, and found myself caught in that inevitable situation that happens when you slam down an extra-large Diet Coke at the beginning of your trip. I thought I could get away with doing the two-hundred-mile journey without making a pit stop, but my bladder didn't stand a chance in the middle of the mountains. I had to pee so badly that it looked like I was pregnant again and felt like I was having contractions! I kept driving . . . and driving . . . and driving. I pulled into a fast-food parking lot in a heart-pounding panic. *I will NOT piss in my own car.* (The big irony here was that I had a brand new box of diapers in my trunk.)

Barely parked, I flung open my door, waddled around my vehicle, and ripped my baby girl out of her car seat. Hunched over and running, holding my girl tight against me (*I will not pee!*), I busted through the glass entrance and went flying into the bathroom. I'd never seen or smelled a bathroom so dirty. Standing in a stall (baby in my arms), I was *this close* to bursting like a broken dam. *The pain* . . . I looked down. Dirty wet floor. Dirty wet toilet paper on the floor. Dirty wet seat covers on the floor. A dirty wet wad of I-don't-know-what-that-is on the floor. I then noticed a nauseating stench rising from the floor. (Just thinking about it makes me gag.) The stall was *disgusting*, but it was my only option.

I looked at my baby. She looked at me. *Crap.* In my mad dash to get to a toilet, I'd forgotten our stroller in the trunk. I had no help, no backup. No countertop, no changing table. Where was I supposed to put my child while I relieved myself on the pot? Trying to fetch the stroller at this point meant pissing in my pants for sure, and I had to get my pants off before I made a bigger mess and turned this awful bathroom even worse. I remember thinking *Just put her on the ground; it'll be good for her immune system.* Then I thought of what my husband would say if she somehow came down with a rare E-coli disease that was traced back to the ladies' restroom floor of that particular fast-food joint. Not an option. I was out of time.

My mind raced. *Move fast,* I thought. With my girl clinging to one of my arms like a hanging monkey and on the verge of major tears, I managed to unbutton, unzip, pull down my jeans inch-by-inch, and cover the toilet seat with one free hand. My heart was pounding with cardio fervor; I was sweating from holding the weight of my baby and how fast I was trying to move. I collapsed onto the toilet, pants successfully down, baby on my lap. *Pssssssssssssssssssssh.* It was the best pee of my life, minus the stench in the stall. I did it. *We did it.* I felt invincible.

My learned lesson that day, besides avoiding extra-large Diet Cokes on road trips? Never underestimate the power you earn from exercising quick problem-solving skills involving babies. Conquering that situation with my daughter, by myself, convinced me that I was capable of pretty much anything that involved motherhood. It was like I had won the New Mommy Olympics.

When you give yourself opportunities to handle mini-emergencies alone, you face certain fears and naturally build your own resilience. I soon found myself problem solving with baby in public places everywhere—changing her diaper on a Styrofoam pad on the floor of Restoration Hardware's storage area when we had an unexpected blowout in the middle of shopping (there were no bathrooms anywhere) and wiping up spilled iced tea on the floor of Crate and Barrel's showroom with spare diapers in my bag (the tea spilled because I had too many shopping bags hanging off our stroller and the whole thing fell backward, with my cup in the cup holder).

I then got greedy and decided to take my grand theory about resilience building through unconventional acts to the next level: I took my girl to a salon. In the name of new mom beauty, I wanted to get a quick pedicure with the expectation that my seven-month-old would sit on my lap the entire time while I got my toes done. Surprisingly, it was a hoot and a half of fun. No, it wasn't impossible. Yes, she did it. And boy, did I wish I'd done it sooner. Here's why you should steal a pedicure with your baby on your lap, too, any time after the four-month birthday and before she starts to crawl:

1. Baby can most likely sit up and is happy sitting on your lap anyway.
2. It's a good excuse to get out of the house.
3. You're probably craving some kind of beauty treatment anyway.
4. Taking a baby to appointments that you don't typically take babies to teaches you trial-by-error tricks and problem-solving skills if and when things get sketchy and baby gets antsy.
5. The sooner you start taking your babe to places where they can "learn to wait," the better. (But bring those toys, just in case . . .)
6. It's fun and funny to watch them bounce on your lap as your toes turn pretty.
7. The pedicurists get a kick out of it.
8. You prove to yourself that you can handle any situation when put in the position. Even if baby cries, the world won't end.
9. Baby learns life skills and social confidence being out with you, in the real world, that you can't teach at home.
10. It's always impressive to see a new mom living life as she did before with baby, especially when the mom is confident doing it.

Just remember: feed babies before venturing out and make sure you go during a time that fits into the wake/play part of their schedule!

The more things you take charge of to create a mommy-and-me team for your day-to-day life as a woman, the more normal your life feels. Just because it's difficult to grocery shop with baby doesn't mean there's not extreme value in it (you learn how to cope with baby in the cart, your baby learns how to be out in the world). Just because most women don't take their kids to quick beauty treatments doesn't mean you can't do it. The more you strip away the fear in tackling small feats with your child, the better you'll be equipped to handle every future situation and the more adjusted your baby will be. Commit to handling far-fetched situations with baby head-on, whether it's peeing with your daughter on your lap or taking your son with you to get a pedicure—it's the best way to declare war on Mommy Brain.

Ditch Your Duties!

While fighting the fabulous fight against Mommy Brain is paramount, you also need to balance your ballbusting by ditching your baby around four or five months—with or without your spouse. Taking a marked break from your mommy duties is a must-add to our postpartum to-do list. (I'm not talking about getting a sitter for a few hours so you can get some air; you should've done that around the one-month mark!) Although I never had any issue leaving my girls with sitters when they were babies, I'd have never attempted to leave town if it weren't for Oscar-winner Matt Damon and his 2011 movie *The Adjustment Bureau*. (Never seen it? Don't fret. Let's just say it wasn't quite in the same category as his *Bourne Identity* movies.) Matt was the push I needed to keep that first bounceback of mine bouncing.

I shouldn't give Mr. Damon all the credit; the brutal truth is that my mom made me do it and used Matt's fame and adorable face to seal the deal. When my first daughter was around five months old, I unexpectedly got a call from a former employer asking if I was available to fly to New York City to interview him for his new movie. I said yes instantly, as I've been conditioned to do thanks to working in entertainment: *just say yes and figure it all out later.* I then almost wimped out and changed my yes to a no thank-you-I-can't-I-just-had-a-baby days later. Enter, My Mom (via telephone).

"You have to go! It's Matt Damon!" she yelled at me on the phone. Without hesitation, my mom told me to toughen up, that she could watch my girl and that I'd better get my butt out of the city so that I could have some valuable time to remember who I was before my daughter busted in. My mom is one of those women who has always been a solid advocate for staying true to yourself after having kids (bar hopping and dancing on tables excluded). She reminded me that I wouldn't have said no to the job before baby, so why would I say no now, especially since I had her to watch my child when I'd be away? (Now that I think about it, she probably concocted this little plan just so she could play fun Grandma with my little girl!)

The trip would literally be for thirty-six hours; fly there, interview the cast, fly back to Los Angeles. I remember the day I left. I worried about traveling so far away when my daughter was so small. I got weird and weepy after I kissed her chubby cheeks, got in the car to head to the airport, and watched her snuggled up as a small bundle in my mom's arms as I drove away from my doorstep and headed to the airport. I questioned my intentions and whether I was doing the right thing. *Would my girl wonder where Mommy had gone overnight? Am I selfish? Is this really worth it?* I felt all the first-time clichés that happen with most mothers when we leave our babies for an extended amount of time: doubt, sadness, longing, guilt. I felt it all, until I demanded to myself that I stop it.

Guilt is a choice; make the choice to opt out. Someone you love and trust very much (and who is much more qualified than yourself) is caring for her. And, your husband is there, for goodness sakes. You're not doing anything bad. It's true what they say about your heart turning mushy when it's time to leave babies for the first time. I let myself feel it, but then I made myself get over it. *Compartmentalize this feeling and be a nondramatic grown-up; this is work, moms work.*

If I had embraced the guilt (like some moms I know suggest to do), I know exactly what would've happened: I would've traveled across the country only to be preoccupied, bomb my interviews, and potentially risk not being hired by this particular employer again. The entire trip would've been a waste of time and money on both sides, and we moms don't have anything to waste. Once I was on the plane, I was fine. Great, even. I was balanced. That trip refreshed and energized me in a way that I didn't even know I needed (and yes, Matt was absolutely adorable and fun and sweet and totally worth the five-minute interview).

My humble recommendation here is to force yourself to do an overnight trip, without your baby, sometime before your child turns six months old. Given that you and your baby are healthy, put it on the calendar and don't overthink it—*just do it*. Waiting past your baby's six-month birthday will only make the goal more distant; the longer you procrastinate something, the more far-fetched the task is to accomplish. Then, if you're like some moms I know, you find yourself exhausted, at your wit's end, and seriously confused about why you can't seem to pull yourself together or away from your kids and get a moment for yourself years later. Small doses of separation are healthy for the overall well-being for moms and babies, even if Matt Damon isn't involved! Go spend the night at a hotel down the street if you have to. Just get out.

Now that you've got "ditch your duties" on your list, let's talk about starting a major endeavor separate from your baby.

Project Motherhood Begins . . .

When it comes to jump-starting focus for life after baby, this section might be the most important part of this book. I urge you to read closely, read thoroughly, read like you really mean it. Starting a project that has nothing to do with your parenting duties or baby's milestones has incomparable potential to bounce your mind back like a real mother. (If you already work, then consider your work already fulfilling this plan.)

What was my project? I started blogging—and it turned into something that I single-handedly credit for uplifting my postbaby spirit, making me feel like me again, and reinventing my career for the long run. While your future project may be something totally different and unrelated to anything I describe here, I'll use my experience to detail what I developed and how it helped me.

The absurd notion of starting a new and unfamiliar project, as I was becoming a first-time mom, came from my single, child-free, social media genius friend Shira Lazar (founder and host of the digital series *What's Trending*). You remember my frank tale at the beginning of this book, when I cried for most of my pregnancy, for fear I'd never accomplish career goals again after my first baby was born? I went to lunch with Shira a few weeks before my due date and told her about it. "You should start a mom blog," she told me with this crazy look in her eye over lunch in a hipster Holly-wood neighborhood, sitting outside in the summer heat, me with a nine-month-pregnant belly hanging over my chair. I just looked at her blankly.

"I don't know anything about blogging," I said. Truth was, I barely knew how to use email and was only on Facebook because the marketing department at my previous employer (cable network ReelzChannel) had started a profile for me, as I was one of their on-camera hosts. I barely knew how Facebook worked, and you bet I wasn't even remotely interested in finding out what the hell the then-brand-new Twitter thing was all about. (Instagram? It wasn't even around yet.) "I'm telling you, start a blog," she repeated. This was a young woman whom I'd teased for joining Twitter so early on yet also admired her because of her foresight, creativity, tenacity, and ultimate hustle in the media world. *Just do what Shira says*, I thought.

Writing was always a serious love of mine (since writing my very first "book" in the sixth grade about two sisters named Leanne and somebody else, I can't remember), but technology had never been my thing. How do you even start a blog? With my due date weeks in front of me, I knew my free time was limited, so I got on it quick. That afternoon, I went home and Googled "mom blog." Then, I Googled "how to start a mom blog."

The world opened up with websites, forums, chat rooms, resources, and everything that existed in the mom blog world back in 2009. (Keep in mind, the blogging world back then was nowhere as developed or half the branded industry it is now.) I started clicking and reading and following and clicking some more. I had a little less than twenty-one days to figure out this budding industry before my baby decided to kick herself out and turn my world upside down. My husband was suspiciously on board with it. "Yeah! You should start a blog!" he'd tell me.

A few days later, I got a text from Shira: *There's a speaker panel about mom blogs happening at this summit I'm speaking at . . . you should go.* I got the info and found myself in an unfamiliar space the following week, now with a belly that was literally days away from my due date. I listened to the speakers and read their bios; these were seriously accomplished women who were famous for being pioneers in the blogging space for moms.

After the panel, I walked to the head of the room in my stretchy pants and long tank top (I was wearing some smokin' platform sandals, though). My heart pounded. I think my belly pounded. I was sweating. I'd never felt so out of my league in my life. I approached the moderator of the event, famed blogger Jessica Gottlieb, and introduced myself in a wavering voice that made me feel like I was fourteen all over again.

"Hi! I'm Jill. I'm a TV host and am starting a blog right now and was wondering if you have any leads I might be able to reach out to in the 'new mom' space . . . a website I might be able to start writing for, to get my feet wet?" Jessica looked down at my belly, paused with what I assume was complete confusion, and then up at me. *She thinks I'm crazy, coming here ready to pop, inquiring about job opportunities.* (If you know Jessica and her deadpan sarcasm, you might be cackling at what you imagine her expression might've looked like in that moment.)

She smiled and was wonderful. "There's a web series called *Momversation* that might be interesting for you. You should reach out to Jennifer Brandt, she's the managing editor. Here's her email address." And then she gave me Jennifer's email address. I went home and hit my email right away, writing to this "Jennifer Brandt," explaining my new goals in the digital space and what kind of deadline I was on to get involved—you know, with an impending due date and all.

Long story short, Jennifer wrote a most positive and friendly note back and gave me a few pointers about the hows and whats of blogging. (So you know, Jessica and Jennifer have boosted me up to this day. . . . I consider them some of my most treasured professional friends.) My baby girl was born about a week later, and I started writing about my own strange experiences as a new mom during my newborn's naptimes on Tumblr (which was brand new at the time). I soon jumped into joining and learning the rhythm of Twitter, by trial and error, and began interacting with as many mom-bloggers as I could find during my little lady's snoozes. After a few months of watching and stalking online trends and standards, I started searching for a solid domain name I could develop into a real blog of my own.

Every domain that felt remotely relatable to me, catchy names that I connected to, was taken. I searched more. I typed every URL possibility I could think of and then plunked out variations of it to make sure I hadn't missed a domain that was available. After about thirty minutes of hardcore searching, cursing, and dropping all kinds of F-bombs, it happened: *TheFABMom.com is available!* I bought it without a thought. I hired a designer for five hundred dollars, told her what looks and colors I liked, and had myself a blog. TheFABMom.com went live on February 1, 2011 (my first birthday after becoming a mom) and became my instant, second baby. I call this time in my life The Great Career Bungee Jump.

During my real life baby's two naps per day through her first year, I'd sit down at my computer and write, click, read, and educate myself like a rogue about the digital world. I wrote blogs and hit publish. (I got in trouble with my husband for writing some of them, which I then deleted out of wanting to stay married.)

I researched resources and sent blind emails to popular bloggers and digital video companies asking if I could pick their brain or write guest posts for them. I made BIG mistakes that, looking back at now, I still can't believe I made and am embarrassed about. But I kept going. I had a naptime project to tend to (between throwing in loads of laundry and emptying the dishwasher) that had nothing to do with my baby; something that kept me productive, creatively thinking, and feeling like my prebaby hustling self. I fed on the adrenaline of occupying my thoughts away from baby while she was asleep and became focused in a most shocking way. I ultimately found myself happier and more present when my daughter was awake.

Starting my project—my blog—forced me to feel bold, have confidence in myself, and committed to learning something outside of motherhood that fulfilled me as a woman, which energized me as a mom. It doesn't matter if you decide to make bracelets, read *Gone with the Wind* for the fourth time, study for your broker's license, or chip away at an application to finally apply for medical school while your baby sleeps—just pick something that floats your boat and *do* it. Commit to something separate from your baby, an activity that goes beyond motherly duties and requires your brain to engage on an adult level. If I can do it, you can do it. Feeling like a useful, evolving grown-up is a cornerstone of human happiness, so trust this will also enhance your stamina as a mother in the long run. (Because it will.)

CHAPTER 8

YOUR BABY BODY

By this time, you're either amazed at how the hell the baby weight did indeed fall off or cursing why the hell it hasn't seemed to fall off at all. Either way, you must continue to pay special attention to your body through baby's first year without getting frustrated.

A study published by Public Library of Science (PLOS) in 2016 cites a connection between new moms gaining too much weight between pregnancies and possible harm to the next baby coming down the pipe (or tube, I should say). They found that moms who gained between 8 to 9 pounds or more between pregnancies had a 33 to 78 percent increased risk of their next babies having a low Apgar score (a measure of newborn health), neonatal seizures, and meconium aspiration (when a baby inhales his waste and amniotic fluid before or during birth), as compared with moms whose weight was stable between pregnancies. Granted, these finding had all sorts of questionable variables, but a study is a study, and I am mentioning it here for informational purposes only.

Shedding postbaby weight is personal and does not determine anyone's value as a mom or woman (hello, we already know that!), but whether we lose it can also (unfortunately) influence how we feel about ourselves only because we may not feel like "us" with extra pounds that are there because of having a baby. Blame impossible media standards or plain and wrongful judgment and pressures against women, but you and I know that old habits die hard.

No matter where you are in your postbaby weight journey around your child's six-month birthday, you must keep moving. Whether we opt to do thirty-minute walks with our babies in strollers or take part in mommy-and-me fitness programs via local groups, apps, video streaming series, or DVDs, one thing remains true: a gym is not necessary for new mom exercise! The sooner we grasp that, the quicker the body and mind bounces back.

Naked bathroom fitness?

After my second daughter, I rarely got to the gym. I still don't get to the gym more than once every few weeks at the time of this writing—that's the bitter truth. Genetics play a major part in how fast baby weight comes off, and for whatever reason, my genes somehow kept me slim between babies. (If it balances the scale any, I bump up my nonexistent bustline with absurdly padded bras and fool television viewers into thinking I actually have a nice mane of hair on my head with extensions. Feel better?) But seriously, how did I maintain moderate fitness after babies? I got naked.

In my twenties, I used to watch television while doing sit-ups in the name of keeping a fit figure—yeah, that stopped happening once I had kids. After motherhood, the rare opportunity to actually watch television became something that I most certainly did *not* want to ruin by doing push-ups! How would I be able to pick apart every expression and catty comment on the *Real Housewives of Beverly Hills* if I was distracted with getting my exercise on? Post-babies, I came up with another plan.

At night, in my bathroom, it was *on*. I stripped down, shut the door, and got down to business for about ten minutes right before my shower. *Get your mind out of the gutter.* (I mean, yeah, my husband and I did have our fun, as couples do—which explains Baby #2 just nine months after Baby #1 was born. Sex *is* known to also offer great cardio.) But no, I trapped myself naked in my bathroom for the sole purpose of exercising on a daily basis. For me, the keys to staying fit are to make good use of time any way I can and to keep my muscles feeling present.

What do I suggest doing for this naked fitness routine? Here's what worked for me:

- *Push-ups against the bathroom sink.*
  I started doing these before I brushed my teeth and quickly lumped them into my preshower routine once I realized I didn't want to get sweaty before brushing my teeth. Doing push-ups against the sink at a forty-five degree angle, rather than getting on the floor to do traditional ones, are much easier but still build strength. Doing two sets of fifteen most every night kept my muscles feeling present.

- *Heel raises to work the calves.*
  Standing up straight and raising heels off the floor into a tippy-toe position work the calves like no other exercise

really can. You can hold onto your sink for balance or suck in your tummy to keep your own balance and up the intensity.

○ *Butt squats.*
My husband always liked to identify this exercise as, "What's the point of that weird move?" Standing with your feet parallel and shoulder-width apart, keep your hands in praying-like position in front of you at your chest (to keep your balance). Suck in your tummy. Keeping your back straight, bend your knees, stick your booty out far (so that you can feel a bit of strain in your buns, and it looks and feels like you're sitting down), and keep bending as far as you can go with your back straight and knees bent directly over your feet. You'll quickly feel the burn in your buns and thighs—at least I did (and still do). Straighten your legs and come back up as fast as you can, squeezing your bottom as you rise up to stand up straight. (Is this even making sense? Damn. I wish I could include a video in here.) Repeat as many times as you can stand it, and as long as your spouse refrains from making fun of you should the door be unlocked.

○ *Touch your toes.*
Stand up, keep your legs straight, bend over from the waist, and just let your body hang there. Breathe. Hang some more. Touch your toes if you can. Feel the stretch up the back of your legs and just relax. If you hold a stretching position for ten seconds or more, it lengthens muscles in a way that keeps you limber, agile, and relaxed from the inside out.

☺ *Stretching arms up as high as they can go.*
Stand up tall with arms stretched all the way up to the ceiling while facing forward, and then lean to one side and then the other.

This entire routine takes no more than ten minutes, which is why I found it conveniently doable before showering. Not to mention, you'll be naked and will most likely get glimpses of yourself doing this vigilante fitness regimen in front of a mirror, which can motivate any woman like a real mother. Something else I did, naked in the bathroom? I took advantage of blow-drying my hair while hanging upside down. You know, to get a deep hamstring stretch. This is multitasking at its best, women; feel the relief in your lower back and enjoy the extra volume in your mane (from drying it upside down). After you conquer your powder room in the nude, you might want to hit the kitchen.

Kitchen Calorie Burning.

I should be transparent and just rename this section for what it is: a call to clean your own home in an effort to burn calories while getting organized and feeling productive at the same time. Yes, exercise can be accomplished via housekeeping if you do it often enough—the bending, the pushing, the wiping, the scrubbing, the reaching. If you do it fast, you've got yourself a legitimate heart-pumping, cardio situation. This absurd and relatively sexist concept hit me one day as I was washing baby bottles at my sink (because, you know, that no-breast-feeding thing).

I hated washing baby bottles. (Then why didn't you just nurse, lady? See chapter 5 again.) Scrubbing bottles and plastic nipples and those pesky two-part filters that supposedly reduce baby's gas consumption while drinking was my most dreaded task at the end of the day. I purposely stocked myself with about eight bottles from the beginning so that I didn't have to constantly wash them. Every day, I'd use them as my baby's schedule was carved: a bottle around 7 a.m., when she'd first wake up, then again at 10 a.m., another at about 1 p.m., one around 4 p.m., and then another at about 7 p.m., which would be the last one before I'd put her to bed. (This schedule was pretty much in full effect from the time my girls were two months old up until their introductions to and mastering of solid foods around four or five months. Then things got easier with more time between feedings and less bottle washing, as you'll soon see.)

Every time I'd stand at my kitchen sink full of hot water and suds and holding that scrubber on a stick, I'd curse the endless washing in my head. *This is a classic case of how mom duties can feel like a waste of time. I wish I was doing something productive right now.* Why didn't I just toss everything into my dishwasher? Well, because my dishwasher at the time wasn't that effective and always left spots and residue all over the clean dishes, and I didn't want that on my baby's bottles. *Wash wash wash, waste waste time.* And then, one night, a light bulb flipped on in my head: suck in your stomach as you wash all the bottles! *Ding ding ding! You've just unwasted your time!*

Ballerinas spend hours sucking in their tummies while they do barre work. Pilates instructors stress the importance of engaging core strength while doing plank poses. Yoga enthusiasts know how imperative it is to hold in one's stomach to maintain balance. Washing bottles quickly became my go-to workout at the end of the day while standing at my sink and getting my baby's bottles ready for the next day of manual mommy labor. I'd stand up straight, suck in my abs (to the point that yes, I did feel a bit sore and winded afterward), breathe deeply, and take breaks as I needed and scrub-scrub-scrubbed. Washing bottles would usually take me around ten to fifteen minutes each night. That's a heck of an abs workout, if you ask me!

What other domesticated duties burn calories while baby naps? Based on an average weight of 150 pounds, the following activities can serve as makeshift workouts:

- *Vacuuming* for 60 minutes burns approximately 200 calories.
- *Cleaning a bathroom* for an hour burns about 180 calories.
- *Gardening* (planting, weeding, digging) has the power to burn 250 calories an hour.
- *Cooking* can burn 150 calories per 60 minutes. (I'm personally convinced this is because of all the standing.)
- *Sweeping and mopping* is a total body workout that can shave 240 calories off if you do it for an hour.
- *Shoveling snow* (yikes!) can burn more than 400 calories in an hour.
- *Ironing* can burn nearly 150 calories if you do it for 60 minutes straight (hello, triceps).
- *Cleaning, dusting, and straightening up* can add up to 170 calories burned per hour.

Just for added motivation, dress yourself in workout wear every day—unless you're actually venturing out and want to look cute or professional, that is. Wearing sneakers and stretch pants has a magical effect of making me feel like I'm exercising throughout the day even if I don't get to the gym (which, like I said, I rarely do these days). I wore my hot pink running shoes and black leggings every chance I was home during the day that first year of motherhood because they physically supported my body to keep moving throughout the day. And, here's an extra FAB tip: set a timer to ring in ten-minute intervals whenever you take on a chore to motivate you to move as fast as you can. I call this tip Instantly Inspired Cardio. Add music and the whole scene gets better. Fun, even, if you remember to stay mindful and keep your mind on what you're doing while tackling your tasks. (Gasp!)

---

3 Fixes for Fitting in Fitness with a Baby in the House

From Jennifer Cohen, mom, author, TV personality, and president of No Gym Required

How's this for honesty: I've never met Jen Cohen in person! However, I have been a fan for a long, long time (we have mutual friends). Jen's savvy longtime philosophy of not needing a gym to exercise has been an idea I've lived my life by the past few years. Heed her tips here.

1. **Schedule a workout, even if it's only for 5 to 10 minutes!** By setting aside a couple minutes for your workout every day, you'll start to rebuild habits and get back into a routine. All it takes is a little consistency, so make your workout time nonnegotiable.
2. **Take advantage of naptime.** While your little one sleeps, find motivation to work out with the furniture in your house. Use chairs, couches, and step stools as your equipment for squats, push-ups, and abdominal workouts. There are also an unlimited amount of apps you can download

---

that have awesome 5-minute workouts (you can even stack them when you have 10 minutes, etc.).

3. **If you can't beat 'em, join 'em.** When finding a peaceful time to exercise seems impossible, include your baby. You can do curl-ups (for thighs) with them sitting on your lap, airplane planks with them laying on your shins (as you lie on your back and work your abs), and more. Mommy-and-me fitness classes are becoming the norm, so check out your options either online or at local gyms in your area. Exercising with baby is actually fun and a great way to bond!

Now that you're toned up and tuned in, it's time to hit the sack . . .

No Babies In Bed!

This is the part of the book when cosleeping advocates come running toward me with flaming torches, demanding and warning all of you to run far, far away from me as soon as possible. Cosleeping has a small share of scientific research that backs it up as being a healthy choice for parents and kids, but it also carries a hefty dose of dangers and warnings, too. (Let's just say the American Academy of Pediatrics' latest recommendation for infant sleep safety, at the time of this writing, instructs parents to NOT cosleep with their babies. I'll let you look this up on your own—too much details for me to get into here.) I make the case to ditch cosleeping simply because we live in a demanding, high-pressure world where sleep is more valuable than ever. Backers of cosleeping will argue it has the power to do a lot of good for babies; I will argue (along with most of today's leading and accredited pediatricians) that cosleeping with your baby has the danger of bringing new parents down fast. And a fast fall doesn't quite make for a big bounce.

To be perfectly frank after babies (there's that f-a-b again), I'll tell you what I did with both my daughters in a quick and glossy way for purposes of saving time: I kept my girls in bassinets, right next to my bed, for the first three to almost-four months of their lives and then moved them to their own cribs in a separate room. I was insistent on teaching them to learn to self-soothe and was a big believer in sleep-training babies when the time was right (usually around four months). To paraphrase what my friend and pediatrician Dr. Tanya Altmann advises, encouraging babies to self-soothe themselves to sleep is the first most valuable skill they are capable of learning as infants. Consult your own pediatrician about the specifics and put it on your must-ask questions for that well visit around the three-month mark.

Did we have hiccups and clashes in our self-soothing and sleeping plans? Of course we did (you will, too!), and in very different ways between my two girls—my firstborn caught on quick and slept in her crib without any issues at all, while my second baby insisted on being cuddled for what seemed more than humanly possible. (My youngest continues to make efforts to force her way into our bed, which I consistently refute and correct, as a four-and-half-year-old at the time of this writing.) While resiliently rolling with the punches my babies socked to me, I stayed dedicated to sleep training. You must too, to bounce back in the long run.

What is sleep training? Sleep training is the process of teaching babies how to soothe themselves so that they fall asleep on their own and stay asleep through the night. Depending on what modern method you choose, sleep training may involve putting a baby down before he dozes off in your arms or letting your baby cry for marked periods of time before you head into the room to soothe them back to sleep. Most methods of sleep training operate on the assumption that your baby is not sleeping in your bed with you, because (duh) there's no training associated with cosleeping— the child simply doesn't know how to go to sleep unless you're in there with him!

Sleeping with your baby can be the most precious experience— trust me, I know. (I'm a sap just like everyone else, despite many things I've suggested in this guide.) I remember the baby smell, I remember pushing my face so close right up to each of my daughters as they lay peacefully on top of my bed because they just looked like little angels up close (and that smell!). I remember the feeling of wanting to savor and squeeze everything because they were so magically tiny. We *should* savor all those things moderately, without forgetting the greater goal to get everyone to sleep independently. We eventually want our babies, toddlers, and older children to sleep healthfully and independently as they grow, for all parties' safety and benefit. Everyone needs his or her own bed. Otherwise, you might start losing your mind when month eight— or year five—rolls around, and your kid is still nudging their foot in your eye, in your bed, at 2 a.m.

Constant cosleeping does not teach infants to fall asleep on their own, nor is it comfortable or safe for everyone involved. Some medical doctors encourage it, some will tell you to get that baby out of your bed—everyone is different, and you'll do what feels right to you as each situation present itself. (I'm just here to tell you how I bounced back, remember?) I guarantee you will cosleep with your babies many times and enjoy it, but it's also up to you to protect your own sleep and not let cosleeping turn into a go-to habit just because it's easier in the short run. Remember, she who works the hardest at establishing a solid foundation wins in the long run. *But my kid can't be sleep trained. I've tried.* Excuse my bluntness, but: you're most likely not trying hard enough. Some kids take more work than others.

These days there is an overabundance of expert sleep information, workshops, and online classes or seminars you can access to help guide you to sleep train your baby. Get some balls and get the job done, somehow, some way. (Balls bounce, remember?) One particular friend of mine refused to let her child whimper or cry when it came to bedtime. "I won't do that," she'd tell me. "Okay," I'd say as I listened to her whine and pine every time we talked about not being able to sleep peacefully, how her child was incapable of sleeping without her (yes, including naps), and how she constantly felt like she was spinning out of control because she refused to get her family's sleep under control.

Don't torture yourself thinking that sleep training will "make your child cry" or that it's just "too hard." Do the right thing. Even my friend Dr. Tanya (from earlier, with the breastfeeding tips) often tells parents that one of the first, most valuable skills a baby can learn is to self-soothe. You can and must figure it out because good and effective parents do what's right for their whole family in the long run, even if there is some crying involved.

On a side note: do you plan to have a sexual relationship with your partner after baby? *Oh yeah, that.* Babies in your bed don't exactly lend to couples rediscovering each other. In a study from Pennsylvania State University published in 2016, 140 parents allowed themselves to be filmed in sporadic, overnight scenarios at home; parents who coslept with their children beyond the baby's age of six months tended to experience varied marital troubles involving adjustment-after-baby, higher family chaos, and a lower quality of putting their baby to bed. In other words, husbands and wives who coslept with kids past the six-month mark seemed to have more family issues than those who opted out of the family bed situation. Researchers were quick to point out that the findings don't indicate cosleeping itself to be negative, but that consistent cosleeping with older babies possibly points to problems in the couple's relationship and/or maternal anxiety that might prompt parents to cosleep with their babies in the first place.

Make an effort to establish healthy sleep habits for your baby, your spouse, and yourself. Pull your big girl panties up and pick a sleep-training method that you can peacefully and purposefully conquer when your baby starts dropping the night feedings between four and six months old. Sleep training is not easy, but set your emotions aside and go at it to get the job done to the best of your ability. Some babies take to it easy (my first child), and some will fight you to the death (my second child). Do your best and find satisfaction that you're doing your best no matter how much or little your baby catches on. Make the effort to succeed in the same way you worked to get that degree, job, or promotion years ago for the sake of your future physical health (i.e., sleep and sex with our partners).

Moving on now to filling up our already-full hearts even more in most unexpected ways . . .

CHAPTER 9
YOUR BABY HEART

Settling in with motherhood is a process that doesn't really stop (as I'm experiencing this myself with my six- and five year-olds). Getting past the newborn stage can feel like reaching the light at the end of the tunnel (yes!), but then you look up and there's another damn tunnel in front of you (hello, toddler years). So you head in there, not sure what to expect, and look for the next light to follow. And then it's Kindergarten (holy mother of how did that happen). You get me? You will.

As entertaining and fulfilling as it is to discover the miracle of growth and development as our babies get bigger, start to smile, sit up, and crawl before our eyes, we also need something for *us*, too. A tangible token that screams *I sought and I conquered* every time we look at it. Remember that chat we had about filling up our own confidence tanks throughout those challenging newborn days? It's time to reward ourselves, so we can remind ourselves how fabulous we are in the most mundane times even if just for moments here and there. Bust out your wallet, it's now time to buy some stuff.

The MOMento

Who thinks "push presents" are ridiculous? Me. Pregnant women everywhere (maybe even you) might now want to gag me and lock me in a closet after reading this. *Shut up, Jill! Women deserve something special and fabulous and sparkly when they become mothers!* We do . . . but here's my wacky, wonderful idea: we should get that special or sparkly memento ourselves, somewhere around six to eight months into the whole motherhood game. Why? It means so much more to earn it and get it later rather than nabbing it right when the baby pops out.

Apparently I wasn't savvy enough to coerce a push present from my husband either time around. I never thought asking for a gift that coincided with the birth of our children was all that important. I mean, if he were to show up with some kind of glittery ornament as an I-love-you-forever-and-ever-and-you're-amazing surprise, hell yes I'd take it—but I never put any kind of push present pressure on him. Yes, pregnancy and childbirth are not a cocktail party. Yes, our lives, minds, and emotions irreversibly evolve after becoming mothers. But no push presents needed, please. Instead, I say we go for something much more meaningful—a concept I've coined The MOMento.

This idea is rooted from when I first started working in television back in 2007. After a few long years trying to break into the oversaturated Los Angeles market as an on-camera talent, I landed my first job as an entertainment reporter with a newly launched cable network called ReelzChannel (heard of it?). I was beyond thrilled and weepy and overly thankful to God and The Universe for somehow allowing my big dream of interviewing celebrities to come true after an embarrassing amount of hard work and too many disappointing runarounds to recount now. After scoring the gig, I wanted to commemorate my luck and accomplishment in a tangible way that would last through my life. My mom came up with a brilliant idea: "Why don't you buy yourself a piece of jewelry?" So, I did.

I window-shopped leisurely to find something special I could see myself loving and living with as I grew older and more mature. I fell for a more-than-what-I-wanted-to-spend ring—a contemporary, silver-and-gold piece with small colored stones that reminded me of the ReelzChannel logo. I was single, childless, and free, so I bought it without regret. *Yippee!* A few years and another job later, I snatched myself another ring in honor of landing a cohosting job with Travel Channel's *America's Worst Driver* (that ten-episode reality show that appeared in a flash and then disappeared just as quickly as it appeared in early 2010). Buying rings soon became my symbol for professional accomplishment. Every time I looked at my decorated fingers, rings on, I felt surges of pride and motivation for pulling certain feats off in my small life and developing career.

After that second ring came a baby, the launch of my blog TheFABMom.com, another baby, few-and-far-between freelance jobs that never really added up to anything, and a whole lot of diaper changing, dishwasher loading, bed fixing, dinner making, child washing, butt wiping, and well, you get it. There were no more rings, mostly because there were no more accomplishments large enough. See, I had rule about when I was allowed to ring-shop: the job had to be a long-term, permanent position. No loosey-goosey freelance gigs or one-offs were worthy of spending money on jewelry (which sucked, since most of my jobs were loosey-goosey freelance one-offs after babies). Rules were rules, and I abided by them.

And then, on one particularly chaotic parenting day in 2012, when my six-month-old daughter was screaming her head off for no reason and my almost-two-year-old was particularly punchy because she didn't like the way I'd cut her sandwiches for lunch, lightning struck me.

Jobs that warrant rings must be long-term, permanent positions.

Motherhood is a long-term position. Motherhood is a permanent position. No job, career surge, or random accomplishment will ever come close to the happiness, pride, sense of achievement, and confidence I will continue to feel throughout my life as a mom. I loaded my daughters into the car and drove to Nordstrom.

With one swift push of my extralong and semiembarrassing double stroller, I glided right over to the jewelry department. I got my toddler a big pink balloon to hold in an effort to keep her content. My baby, tucked in her blanket and sucking on her pink pacifier, kept looking at me like, "What do you think you're doing, lady?" I looked in the glass cases. Nothing. I rolled over to the next case. Nothing. I circled around to the other side and scanned the silver . . . gold . . . rose gold . . . necklaces . . . bracelets . . . watches . . . rings! There they were. My eyes scanned obsessively. Blue stones, green stones, diamonds (yeah right, that was never going to happen), white stones . . . pink stones. There it was. One large, vertical rectangle, pale-rose-colored stone with four silver bands coming out from each side stared back at me. It was fabulous.

My daughters were still happy in the stroller, so I asked the saleswoman if I could see it up close. *Gorgeous!* I tried it on. *Gorgeous!*

I looked at the price. *Holy Mother Oh Crap Wait.* I found myself back at the more-than-what-I-wanted-to-spend place that my first ring offered me. I gave up. I thanked the saleswoman, returned the ring to her, and circled the jewelry cases more. I thought rationally. *It's pink, just like my girls.* The price was not ideal. *I can wear that forever.* If my husband found out that I'd gone shopping and bought some kind of jewelry without even informing or consulting him, I'd be in hot water. *I have money saved from when I was working years ago; he won't even have to know.* The price was expensive, but technically I could afford it without irresponsible issue. *This ring can be a symbol of conquering back-to-back new motherhood over the past two years.* I rolled us back to the saleswoman and bought it before I could talk myself out of the purchase.

I instantly felt idiotic and reckless. *What did I just do? I have two small children now. Why am I buying myself nice jewelry when we've got to save money for college and life and shoes for these little people's feet that won't stop growing?* With my receipt, my ring, and a pit in my tummy, I pushed my long stroller out of the glass doors and toward the parking garage. I figured I could sort out my confusion and decide whether to take the ring back days later in the privacy of my own home.

Suddenly, I practically ran my girls right into Lawrence Zarian, TV's "Fashion Guy" from ABC's *LIVE with Kelly,* Hallmark Channel, and local Los Angeles news station KTLA (Lawrence and I were briefly acquainted because we both worked in television and are Armenian). It was the first time I'd seen him since becoming a mom. We said hi, I introduced him to my daughters, and then we parted ways. I thought of my previous years working on television and took the random run-in as a sign that buying my ring that day was the right thing to do.

I never hesitated to commemorate my accomplishments as a single woman, so why was I now beating myself up for celebrating mom-life as I'd handled it up to that point? Becoming a mother is the most permanent job a woman will ever have. Thinking of all that diaper changing, dishwasher loading, bed fixing, dinner making, child washing, butt wiping, and blog creating made me realize I'd managed, earned, and learned so much. Rewarding yourself with a tangible MOMento around the six-month mark—a ring, watch, special piece of art, or anything that you look at day in and day out, something that makes your heart skip—will keep you giddy and reminiscent of all the great stuff you've done as a mother so far and motivate you to bounce past parenting challenges as you experience them going forward (at least, that's what my ring has done, and still does, for me). Now you try. Don't worry, I won't tell your spouse.

Give, Make, Love ...

Make love? Did somebody say make love? Slow your roll, honcho. This part's not about that. (Although that is a surefire way to get the heart pumping; feel free to do that as much as you'd like during these baby months leading up to the first year.) The fact is, unless you're back to work around this time of your baby's life, you might start feeling more isolated and detached from the world than you did during the newborn days. The human heart is programmed to connect, to contribute, to feel all the feels that make us feel, well, human. It's your responsibility to chase those things alongside your baby.

What did I find to make my heart extrahappy? Giving. Particularly, giving away clothes. When my firstborn was around six months and I was deep into mostly-stay-at-home-with-a-few-random-jobs-here-and-there status, I kept finding myself looking at my professional career outfits from years past. Seeing them hanging in my closet, literally collecting dust, made me uneasy and sad. They stared at me as if to say, "C'mon lady, you know you're not going to use us like you used to for a while . . . if ever again" (given my choice to take a step back from career after baby). I could feel the six-month slump sneaking into my emotions, and I hated it. *I will not lose my bounce.* But I was at a loss for how to bounce back my spirit.

Thanks to an unexpected charity drive that popped up in my email inbox around that time (led by Los Angeles famous news-woman Wendy Burch of KTLA, who has since become a FAB mom of an adorable baby boy), I piled a ton of my smart blazers and snappy dresses into shopping bags to donate to women getting back on their feet after domestic struggles or substance abuse. I loaded my then-baby daughter (my firstborn) into my SUV and drove to the station. The second I handed my bags over to Wendy (to distribute to the organization she was doing the clothing drive for), something magical washed over me: fulfillment. *I'd never meet these women, but my clothes just might give them the extra spirit and motivation to score a job and get them out of a rut.* (A thought that, ironically, got me out of mine.) Helping another mom becomes a most precious venture when you become a mom. I soon tackled my baby's closet.

Okay, let's be reasonable here—you probably don't want to give away every piece of clothing your baby outgrows, as you most likely want to save stuff for your next potential child (like I did). Or you might have an inkling to stash certain sentimental outfits away for the purpose of accidentally rediscovering them later so you can weep nostalgically about your five-year-old's baby years just by pulling out an old outfit they wore to their first birthday (like I've done).

Since your infant grows like a little weed, though, you'll inevitably find yourself with drawers of crumpled onesies, outgrown hats for newborn heads, too-small pants that once seemed so big, and random pairs of socks. If you're like me, you might also find stacks of rarely used baby blankets that somehow multiplied in the hall closet while you were writing thank-you notes to the friends and family who gifted them to you. Pick a few items you can part with and donate them to a local charitable organization for new moms and babies. And don't forget to take your baby with you when you make the trip to drop everything off.

Giving, without expecting anything in return, is one of life's most surprisingly fulfilling actions. As any new mother will tell you, your heart swells up a few sizes after becoming a mom; apparently it's one of the lasting side effects of childbirth. Suddenly, every circumstance, social cause, or community matter that involves the quality of family life trumps everything else. The reality that mothers and babies from all backgrounds often share the same love for our children and parenting struggles becomes blatantly clear almost instantly.

I found myself giving goods to various organizations several times during my babies' first years: donating things like extra diapers we got too big for before we were able to use them, that extra package of unopened maxi-pads I'd bought before going to the hospital, that bottle of sterilizer I used just once (hey, just because I didn't use it doesn't mean that someone else wouldn't). Every time I donated, my heart felt fuller and more resilient to the petty challenges I was dealing with at home with kids . . . and yours will, too.

What else do you need to actively keep tabs on as your baby grows into his first year of life? Friends. Yes, you need friends . . . and you'd better find them, get them, and keep them, fast. Post-partum support is perhaps the most important factor for making a mom feel secure in her new role. Actress and famous mom of two Mila Kunis fessed up to me at the press interviews for her 2016 hit movie *Bad Moms* about how her girlfriends are *the* driving force to boost her up when she has new-mom breaking points: "I really do think having a group of friends is so important. . . . I have an amazing husband, an amazing family, but I so rely on my group of girls."

For me, I was the first of my circle friends to have a baby (no wonder I was scared!), so I know how it feels to be in the middle of something that all of your favorite people don't really understand. Having friends without children proved to be a double-edged sword. On one hand, they reminded me of the gal I was before motherhood and made the prebaby world still seem close and relevant in my new spit-up world. On the other hand, seeing them reminded me of how "unfree" I'd become. While maintaining my prebaby friends, I also sought out other mothers—new friends—in an effort to surround myself with women who understood where I was at in my life.

Those who know me personally know that I didn't enroll in any Mommy & Me music groups or Baby & Me fitness classes with either of my daughters, but man, did my world open to unexpected friendships when I became a new blogger back then. Suddenly, I found myself at the most fun mom-centric events thanks to Andrea Fellman (original founder of SavvySassyMoms.com, who since sold it to a pair of fab friends who now run the site), at trendy toddler-centric hot spots for group playdates thanks to Momangeles.com, and attending educational fairs with swoon-worthy swag thanks to Los Angeles's Club MomMe and Pregnancy Awareness Month. (That swanky Rosie Pope store opening that I described earlier, the one where I wanted to gush and spill all my belly wrap fangirl secrets to Brooke Burke-Charvet, also falls into this category.) With each event I trotted to (often with my baby), I connected with women who were on my same wavelength.

The ongoing blogger events of Southern California became my unofficial mommy groups that kept my spirits happy during a time of dramatic, personal transition associated with becoming a mother. At the very least, go park yourself on a bench at a local playground and see who else shows up to make casual conversation with. Enroll in a local Parent Education class, just for the social perks. There are even smartphone apps to help you meet like-minded moms in your area (that's a shout to the amazing MomCoApp.com). Nobody hangs out on their front lawn anymore with kids (although I did by myself in those early days), so you've got to go out and find that village of moms like you with similar interests if you want to thrive. No one's going to knock on your door and ask you to play if you don't get out there first.

I'm not suggesting you trade your old friends in for new ones (although that might come later as motherhood changes certain behaviors you're able to socially tolerate from peers; that's a whole other book), but make an effort to initiate new friendships as you make your way through this first year with baby. A wide variety of relationships that feed different parts of your soul—the pre-baby you, the new mom you, and the type of mom you'll eventually settle into—are absolutely key to staying resilient through change. Being able to bounce effectively through the changes of motherhood has a tendency to make you love and respect yourself more . . . and, more love and respect for yourself is always good for baby.

Look Back to Move Forward?

I'll never forget when I first figured out the power of looking back to successfully move forward—it was thanks to my first-born violently vomiting all over our carpet.

I was single-handedly trying to pack our new family-of-three's lives in boxes and bags to move into our first home the next day, and the weeks leading up to the big move had been physically stressful and emotionally depleting. I've never been able to adjust to change quickly, even if the change is good (you recall the unexpected pink plus sign, yes?), and between mom-ing, working part-time jobs, coordinating sitters, signing so many damn escrow papers, and all the everyday things that can drag any new mom's energy down, I felt like I was going to lose it more than I'd ever lost anything before.

I remember feeling pressure pounding down on me during those days, and I found myself feeling unable to pull out of angry moods as the days passed. At around 10 p.m. on a Wednesday night—the night before our first, big move—my baby daughter projectile-puked a fountain of formula that would make Linda Blair in that movie *The Exorcist* look like she had just a bit of a spit-up. I broke down in tears, mostly because my husband wasn't home from a long day yet and I was alone, covered in puke, with boxes still waiting to be packed (by me) around me.

As someone who was raised on hearing the words "Just handle it" for every obstacle that came my way (thanks, Mom), I became determined right then to get my brain positive again. I'd been stuck in a negative, overwhelmed mental loop the past few weeks, feeling detached from reality and trapped in a rut of running and calling and texting and emailing and signing to coordinate all things family and moving . . . and I didn't know how to get back to ground zero. So, I cleaned up the puke, wiped my daughter, and continued to pack. I soon found boxes in the back of my closet filled with relics of my prebaby life. With my baby sitting up and looking at me (*Go to sleep, girl!*), I sat on the floor, sorted through the boxes and wept with delight.

All the pressures of mom-ing, working, coordinating, signing, and adult-ing started evaporating into the smell of Lysol I'd just used to clean up the puke. I flipped through old press passes from when I worked red carpet premieres. I found hilarious pictures from college when I thought that wearing a red spaghetti-strapped crop top in the middle of winter (outside) was sexy. I rediscovered old résumés, ones with internships that I'd forgotten I'd even had listed on them. I found and tried on old shoes that I still don't know how I'd worn dancing and not killed myself. I found the guest book that everyone signed from my wedding. There I was, in that box, before I became a "family." I felt surprised, happy, and oddly proud of who I was and who I'd become. I also found myself feeling grateful for life's changes.

We moved the next day, and, from that point on, I made bits of efforts to insert pieces of my prebaby life into my present life to remind myself of accomplishments or joy I'd strived for in years past, because, in some ways, those things were still a part of me. I uncovered my own Miss America contestant crowns (never won Miss California, but came close!) and put them on a shelf in my bathroom so I'd see them sparkling at me every morning. *Reminder, you did this before baby.* I dug up a picture from a previous decade of my girlfriends and me, all dressed in those satin spaghetti-strap blouses before heading to what ended up being a legendary single-ladies' night out in Hollywood, and put it in a place where I could glimpse at it sporadically, smile, and shake my head. I also reached out to former work colleagues to say hello, inquire about what they were doing, and update them about my life (although, now, all we have to do is search Facebook). Reconnecting with my past made me feel rejuvenated and refreshed as a new mom. My prebaby life suddenly seemed relevant again, even during the messiest diaper changes.

I'm not suggesting any of us try to live in the past to seek satisfaction, but actively reminding ourselves what we've strived for, what we've learned, things we've done, and relationships we've had makes us feel reinvented, well rounded, accomplished, and happy. Realizing that you've evolved is beyond valuable—especially when new motherhood can freakishly make us doubt our identities. Hang that miniskirt you could never bear to part with in the front of your closet, just for kicks. Print out and tape an old résumé or diploma to your fridge for a week, just to see it and think, "Hey, that chick's one sharp tack." Send a former boss an email that says, "Just wanted to say hi. How's business?" and then take note of the positive surge that overcomes you when he or she writes back. Soon, you will feel shockingly productive and satisfied with yourself; you might also feel a bit more motivated as a mother.

Remind yourself who you were, and who you still are, to resiliently bounce yourself out of mental ruts when they sneak up thanks to a baby puking or otherwise. Hey, it worked for me . . .

3 Fixes for Feeling Productive as a New Mom

From Samantha Ettus, mom, work-life balance expert, and author of The Pie Life: A Guilt-Free Recipe for Success and Satisfaction

I first met Samantha online, years ago (Twitter, I believe). I clicked on a bunch of her motivational videos for balancing work and life as a mother and thought, *This woman's got it all figured out. . . . I'm following her.* And she does. Since first tweeting with her, and now knowing her as a friendly colleague from whom I often glean advice, I'm thrilled to report how much her insight about attaining goals in life and career (as a mom) has affected and inspired my work-life balance to be better beyond my imagination. Wisdom from Samantha . . .

1. **Understand the Maintenance Years.** Until your youngest child is four years old, you are in the "manual labor phase" of parenting. Let's call these the Maintenance Years. Your job during these years is to maintain your life and career as it was when your child was born, not to leapfrog five levels. If you just stay in the game through these years, you are winning! The Go for It years are right around the corner.

2. **Expect the Imperfection.** Just like a gooey, messy pie, your life is more delicious because it's full and messy. It will be imperfect and you will miss some things and you will mess up sometimes and that is okay. A full life includes many slices, and when you expect and embrace the imperfections, it becomes a lot more enjoyable.

3. **Milk the Moments!** There are no bad days, bad weeks, or bad years; there are bad moments. When you label hard times as bad days or months, you guarantee they will linger longer than necessary. Remember that all challenges are moments (and teaching this to your children as they grow) to create easier lives in the long run. Labeling a 10 a.m. meltdown as a *moment* gives you and your baby the opportunity for the rest of the day to be awesome.

5 FUN FIXES
TO RESTORE, RESET & REFRESH

No matter how fabulous, together, focused, or energetic you may feel during baby's first year, you will have, as our dear friend Samantha Ettus mentioned in the previous section, *bad moments*. (I used to call these times bad days, but Samantha quickly set me straight.) Everyone has bad moments—I did and I still do. Sometimes, I still call my mom to complain about something so stupid and trivial I almost want to slap myself for it. Bad moments might be spawned by your baby refusing to sleep or because you happen to stink thanks to skipping showers for naps. Whatever less-than-stellar moments your days provide, you must restore, reset, and refresh quickly. Here are five fixes to try.

1. *Bake something.* No, this is not some antiquated ploy to turn modern moms into something we're not. However, baking can be more powerful than most of us give it credit for. When I saw my colleague Suzanne Marques, entertainment reporter

for CBS Los Angeles, baking cookies on her Instagram feed literally two weeks after her baby boy was born, I thought, *Get it, woman!* What I didn't know at the time was that Suzanne contracted an infection right after birth and had spent six days in a hospital bed. Suzanne's a tough cookie herself (pun intended), but she had a challenging delivery and fessed up to not feeling like herself after birth. In true tough-cookie form, Suzanne did something about it—she baked. "The light activity, the smells preparing the ingredients, and the aroma soothed my soul," she told me when I asked her what possessed her to get so domestic. "It restored my sense of normalcy and felt like something special for me and my baby—sweets for me, more milk for him!" (Did I mention those cookies were oatmeal? Oatmeal has been known to boost breast milk.) You don't have to be a gourmet baker; you can grab some of those slice-able cookie dough tubes and go to town.

2. **Shower.** *How can I possibly shower if I'm short on time, patience, or energy?* You can. Newborns aren't mobile, so stick a pacifier in your daughter's mouth and wheel her rocking chair into the bathroom so you can keep one eye on her while you bathe if it makes you feel better (this is what I did). If you have a crawler and can't leave them alone for fear they'll get into something dangerous? Put them in their crib with toys or drag that entire pack-and-play into the bathroom. Do whatever you need to do to shower, even if your babe screams at you in protest while you're in there. Five minutes of screaming will not break or hurt your baby, even though you might feel like it, but taking that five-minute shower will change your life that day and beyond.

3. ***Throw a party.*** This sounds counterintuitive if you're feeling out of sorts, but inviting friends over always made me pull it together during the first years of motherhood, which was good for my spirit every time. Hosting guests can be hard work (how many times I cursed my big mouth for inviting friends as I rushed around preparing for them—apologies to my friends for this honesty), but it's always worth it. Playing hostess requires you to clean your home, hide the baby gear, and work toward a goal. (Will you finally make that new pasta salad recipe?) What kept my mind active the most included hosting Thanksgiving dinner, impromptu brunches for my girlfriends, and couples' dinner parties on our patio—all while my babies were babies. Seeing folks having fun *in your space* gives you a fresh perspective about how your home still belongs to *you* (rather than all that baby gear) and how you've still got it (even though you have to empty that Diaper Genie in the morning). It's also a blast of a good time!

4. ***Take a vacay.*** (No, I'm not drunk as I write this.) Yes, it is possible to take a trip with a baby! Although I had a strict no-planes rule when my daughters were babies, I did manage to plop them in the car from the time they were two months old for road trips—sometimes with my husband and sometimes solo to visit my parents two hundred miles away. Leaving your home base with your child for an extended amount of time is a lot to handle, but I happen to think it's worth it when you feel the look-what-I-pulled-off rush after it's done. Set your limits by car or go all-out like my friend Evelyn Taft, weather anchor at KCAL/CBS Los Angeles: she loaded up her new family and went to Hawaii a couple months after having her first baby.

"After a rough C-section and baby blues, it was a huge turning point for my mind, body and soul. . . . We ended up going back when our second was three months old. Traveling with two kids was insane, but it helped me bounce back; I started working out again, the babies started sleeping, and we got to spend some amazing quality time as a family." *Aloha* to that.

5. ***Lunch (with wine) by yourself.*** Maybe this is something that works for me because I always enjoyed my alone time prebabies? (Says the woman who still gets giddy if I find myself alone in my own house for more than an hour's time.) I remember a few specific breaking points during both my daughters' first years, times when I felt suffocated by mommy duties and underappreciated in the wife department, where I just bailed while my husband was at home. I announced I'd be missing in action for an hour and head to a local restaurant to sit by myself, eat in peace, and sip a glass of wine. I didn't go anywhere fancy, I just *went*. I always needed alone time to feel centered before having kids, so I make an effort to maintain that part of my life when needed. Going to the gym, window-shopping, or meeting up with friends can certainly reset us when we're off, but sometimes sitting sans company with a plate of pasta and a glass of Pinot does the trick, too.

Nice try, Jill. These are all fine and fabulous, but hardly rooted in real life and doable for most women. The thing is, they are doable, because real women have done them and lived to tell. Yeah, it can be a lot to handle, but my advice is: *don't think, just do.* Sometimes, the thought of doing something can seem harder than the task actually is. Rise up, forge ahead, get it done. In the words of the incomparable Lucille Ball, "The more things you do, the more you can do." You can't argue with that, especially when it's so darn motivating for new motherhood. If all else fails, make yourself smile—the muscles used to turn your mouth into a grin trigger and release positive endorphins and natural painkillers as you flex them. Say cheese and feel better.

PART 5
STAYING FOCUSED
FOR GOOD

"You have to remember, I'm an autonomous woman who needs friends, and wants friends, and I need to be a wife, so have a date night. You have to remind yourself of how to put your gas mask on first."
—Kristen Bell, mom, actress, and activist

Now that I've dished all sorts of wacky experiments to coincide with caring for a new baby, I'll ask: how do you feel about my suggestions? Do they sound like a hoot or a load of crap that will soon make you flush this book down the toilet? (I sure hope it's not the second option . . .) Here's the hitch: the tips I've offered are solely for the purpose of keeping your mind and spirit focused on things separate from your role as a mother. Staying busy with alternative to-dos will make you feel productive during a time when many new moms find themselves feeling stuck in a black hole of shifting priorities and uncertain identity.

Regardless of your personal beliefs or religious affiliation, consider the old expression: "Idle hands are the devil's workshop." If you allow yourself to get sucked down into the challenging moments of new motherhood without organized distractions (like the ones I've described in this book), it becomes increasingly hard to pull yourself up and out of that pit later. Like I said in the beginning of this adventure: developing resilience has been scientifically identified as a consistent course of action involving:

- *Facing things that scare you.* Leaving baby with childcare, even if you don't feel like you're ready.
- *Developing an ethical code to guide daily decisions.* Being organized each day; starting with making your bed by 10 a.m.
- *Building a strong network of social support.* Making new friends or throwing that party at your house with old friends.
- *Making physical exercise a habit.* Leg squats in the nude before a shower, anyone?
- *Developing mindfulness.* I will only think of washing bottles while I'm washing bottles . . .

Is it all coming together now? We're almost there. Let's bounce a bit more . . .

CHAPTER 10
FAILING FORWARD & FEELIN' IT

The first year with baby brings changes, joy, questions, concerns, and more love and happiness than you would've ever imagined . . . and, there will be fails. *But, Jill! You told us to not ever use the word fail!* Here's another catch: you can, in fact, identify mishaps, bad moments, and random what-in-the-world-was-that experiences only after you've mastered the ability to bounce back from those misadventures with humor and resilience—which is why I'm going to share some of the most epic fails and feats for you to find comfort in on your own journey.

Low Days & High Heels.

To reach the highs, we must first bounce through the lows. (Apologies for being a buzzkill.) Some lows will be silly, some might feel scary or shameful, hopefully none will be too serious in your journey. I always find it helpful to hear about other parents' oopsies in times of trial and doubt, so I'll share a bunch of my own and some famous moms' fails here with you here—you know, to ease the future blows. My first and biggest low was a thing that most new mothers dread ever happening: my daughter rolled off the bed when she was around five months old.

One afternoon when my husband was at work, I laid my girl down smack in the middle of our guest room's double bed to change her, turned and leaned my body for literally seconds to grab a new outfit, turned back toward her and . . . she was on the ground! She didn't cry; she just silently seemed to slip down to the carpet and was looking up at me, shocked. I completely flipped out. Never before did I feel such a mutant strain of panic and fear rush through my veins than at that moment (and the times that followed in future years when this same daughter fell out of her high chair and then accidentally ran into a patio pole while playing with her cousins, or when my younger daughter slipped while learning to walk and cut the back of her head on the corner of my nightstand. I could go on but I'll stop).

Back to the slipping off the bed. The more I remember myself thinking, *I took my hands off her for one second*, the more I wanted to punch myself for sounding like an idiot-cliché. Thankfully my daughter was okay, but I wasn't. Days before this incident happened, a friend of mine had confessed how impressed she was with my "confidence and ease" as a first-time mother, and my head had swelled bigger than it ever had before. *I'm a fabulous mom, even other people think so!* Did my big attitude fool me into feeling untouchable and exempt from messing up? Maybe.

I had flashbacks about other parents' conversations I'd over-heard and judged since becoming a mom: the women in the salon talking about how their kids fell off the couch, the dads who took their kids for a bike ride and returned home with a small broken arm. Hearing those tidbits I'd always think, *Well, why weren't you watching them?* This time it was *me*. Talk about a wakeup call. Even though my girl was luckily unharmed, that first fall took me down hard. I cried, felt guilty, cried more, and really became hysterical when I fessed up the story to my husband days later. He just stared at me and said, in a rightfully irritated tone, "I need to know if stuff like that happens." I started questioning my capability being home with her all day.

Although things are our responsibility and we must stay vigilant when keeping an eye on our children, know this: things happen when babies and kids are concerned. Be as present and aware as you can possibly be and don't be fooled that you're exempt from a bad moment happening when you least expect it. Fails happen to the most FAB, too; deal with them as they come, move forward without fear, and *fail forward* (with more knowledge and experience) so the same thing doesn't happen again.

Not all fails will be serious like my first major one. Most fails will make you feel totally inadequate and then cause you to smile or laugh when you think about them days, weeks, or even years later. The world might feel like it's crumbling down because you can't seem to open your stroller fast enough in a parking lot, in the pouring rain, with a line of cars honking behind you to hurry up and one guy flipping you off (true story). Or, you might feel like a real jackass in the middle of a department store when you take your hands off that same stroller for a second and the entire thing falls backwards—with your baby in it—because you've hooked too many shopping bags on the back (simultaneously splashing your extra-large passion fruit iced tea, which had been in the cup holder, all over the shoe aisle—another true story, thank you very much). There might also be a time when you head to the grocery store, fill an entire cart to the rim with a screaming baby perched in the front basket, wanting the pacifier you accidentally forgot, get to the checkout and then realize you left your wallet sitting on the kitchen counter when the clerk asks you how you'd like to pay (that may've been the worst—I still can't look that guy in the face to this day). Breathe through it all and think, *bounce*.

It also helps to know that famous moms go through the same kinds of fails as you and I. Ali Landry once confessed in an interview with me that, with her first born, she and her husband literally ripped off a gas station pump by accident. "My daughter started to cry in her seat, so I just got in the car [while we were pumping gas] and leaned over her to nurse because I didn't want to take her out of the seat. My husband got in the driver's seat, assumed we were done pumping, and then turned the car on and pulled away from the pump . . . with the pump still attached to our car! We went back to the station to return the ripped-off pump and our hundred-dollar gas cost turned into about a thousand-dollar bill for the broken pump. I felt so bad." See, these new mom mishaps even happen to drop-dead gorgeous actresses and former Miss USAs. Don't ever be embarrassed; just remember to bounce.

For me, bouncing past fails required some kind of visual—a symbol of some sort. I unexpectedly found my symbol in the middle of January a few months after my first daughter was born, on a day I was feeling particularly dumpy and un-bouncy. I was pushing my stroller through Nordstrom, dressed in my go-to black stretch pants and my old pink sneakers. I stopped dead in my tracks when I saw the most eye-popping stilettos displayed on the sale rack in front of me: four-inch, open-toed heels with a big fluffy hot-pink flower puffball on top. That puffball caught my eye and the little voice in my brain screamed, "Buy them! They'll reverse the unfabulous feeling you have now!" So I did.

The heels were irrational and completely off-season, but I felt it was important for me to take a stand and make them mine right then and there. As fabulous as those shoes made me feel (they were my first "for-me" purchase after becoming a mom for the first time), they pretty much chilled in the box, in the bag I brought them home in, in my closet, for the next few months. "I'll wear them when the weather gets warmer," I told myself. Cut to the end of March: the hot pink puffballs were still living in the box.

One particularly uneventful Friday afternoon (those heels still untouched in my closet), I fell into another I'm-not-in-the-mood-for-anything-today mode and threw on my jeans, a long and loose sweater, and running shoes. *Not cute sneakers, running shoes.* I ran some errands with my daughter and ended up back at Nordstrom. I popped into the Ladies' Lounge to feed and change my baby when I saw the scene that remains imprinted in my mind forever. A brand-new mom with a two week old baby (I know because I asked her) was sitting on the couch nursing and decked in skinny jeans, an off-the-shoulder blouse, and open-toed stilettos with straps that wrapped halfway up her leg. *Hot damn.* I was thoroughly amazed and impressed; it was like I had seen a unicorn or something. That new mom in her date-night-worthy outfit sitting with a newborn reinvigorated me that day. She also reminded me that I'd bought some smokin' shoes a few months before.

I went home and walked around my kitchen in my hot-pink puffballs for about thirty minutes. High heels had always and instantly made me feel smarter and more fun because I associated them with work and play, two things that seemed to lessen once I had my first baby. *Ah, yes, I'd forgotten what this felt like.* I took note of the feeling and also took things a few steps further as weeks passed. I started wearing heels once a week—even if the only opportunity was a five-year-old's Saturday morning birthday party at one of those indoor playgrounds. (Yes, I really did wear them to a five-year-old's party.)

Stilettos don't solve big problems, but most of our lows as new moms come from a lot of insignificant constraints that build up over time. Because we tend to get ourselves in a repetitive mom-mode, we don't always know how to let those little things go. Finding a quick and shallow fix—like a pair of stilettos with hot-pink puff-balls to live in your closet—can keep you laughing inside your head and bouncing forward through your most trivial fails that aim to bring you down. I still have these heels in my closet to remind me to "bounce" every time I see them. I haven't worn them since that five-year-old's party years ago, but I don't necessarily need to wear them anymore; they already got me where I needed to go, mentally. Particularly when it came to bouncing through career bumps . . .

Bring Baby to Work?

One of my more memorable fails happened when my mom duties first crashed with career responsibilities. A frenzied day required me to think quickly, problem-solve resourcefully, and also realize that colleagues who truly care about me *will* have my back, especially if that colleague is a mother. Who was the unlikely character responsible for the anxiety I dealt with on this famous day? The wildly talented and raunchy-mouthed actor-comedian Russell Brand (you know, that guy who was married to Katie Perry a long time ago).

My daughter was barely three months old, and I'd started working freelance again—which, in show business talk, means "say yes to every possible job offered to you and figure out the details (i.e., childcare) later." I'd been asked to interview the stars of the then-upcoming movie *The Tempest*, an artsy onscreen reinvention of Shakespeare's classic play. Academy Award winner Helen Mirren was among the cast with Oscar nominee Djimon Hounsou and . . . Russell Brand. I was thrilled. It wasn't expected to be a blockbuster film, but I didn't care—I still had one foot in the career game and was back to talking to celebrities, baby! My interviews were scheduled to happen first thing in the morning, so I booked a sitter until 12:30 p.m.

I headed to Beverly Hills' Four Seasons hotel on the day-of and chatted with Dame Mirren and Djimon right on time. However, the interviews for Mr. Brand seemed to be running late. I waited with the rest of the press in the holding suite. We all killed time catching up, snacking on the chocolate chip cookies, and drinking more coffee to stay alert for when Russell was ready for us. By now, it was almost 11 a.m. *Where is he? My sitter has to jet by 12:30!* Just as I started counting minutes, one of the public relations reps came into the room. "Mr. Brand has to unexpectedly step out for a bit," he said. "He'll be back after lunch for your interviews." *Oh no you didn't, Mother F—er, Russell.* This was a disaster.

I wanted to cry and die of humiliation when I was obligated to explain needing to leave the premises so that I could relieve my sitter. *How embarrassing.* Thanks to one particular friend I had at the movie studio prebaby, who happened to run the press days, I got permission to go home, pack my daughter's things, and bring her back to the interviews with me—she was the one who came up with the idea. "Don't worry, I'll watch her," she said. She was a mom, too; she got it. I went home and later returned with my baby, rolled her into the Four Seasons, through the valet, the elevator, the hallways, and into the holding suites. I was nervous and mortified for being "that mom" who takes her child to work without respect or consideration for professional environments. This was my first significant return to my work scene, and there I was, pushing a baby in a stroller. I had no other choice, so I did it.

To my shock, my girl was quite the hit. "You had the baby! She's so cute! Congratulations!" went on and on, followed by usual questions and sweet stories about their own babies (who were appropriately at home with a sitter, unlike mine). Turns out, most of them told me stories about having to take their kids to work at one time or another, too. I felt so relieved. The gracious friend who offered to watch my daughter in the first place quickly scooped her up out of her stroller, and I headed into Russell's room to meet him.

"Izzat yoh bay-bay out theh in za hallway?!?" Russell leaned in and semi-demanded from his chair the second I walked in and sat down across from him. He had a thick British accent, and his hair was every which way and looked like it hadn't been washed in about seventeen days. (Dare I joke he looked like he'd just had a baby the other day. I say this with the utmost fascination.) I suddenly got nervous. "Yes, it is," I answered. *Don't lose it now, Jill, you've come too far.* He looked confused. "Huh," he replied and then sat back. There was a long and awkward pause, and then I started asking questions. The rest of the interview went fine, minus his delirious gaze. I did my job to the best of my ability that day, retrieved my baby, said good-bye and thank you to my colleagues, and then rolled my stroller back to the valet parking and headed home.

Besides learning the smarts to book a babysitter all day when I get called in for jobs, what was the big lesson? I learned to own my motherhood in my place of work. Becoming a mom gives us added dimension—at home and at the workplace—and that's a powerful thing, no matter what kind of policy your company has about family leave! Your colleagues and superiors will most likely view you as more mature with a baby, so use that opportunity to show how capable you are to handle any situation in a cool and collected way.

Having kids gives us added depth as problem-solvers, which is a positive trait for any kind of workplace—don't forget that. That was the first time I felt equal-parts mother and career woman, and it was because I was forced to collide and control both of my worlds. This fail permanently affected how I started handling mom versus career duties; it gave me added confidence that I could problem-solve my way out of anything, even if there was no other choice than to bring my baby along to get the job done.

My former colleague Orly Shani (style expert for Hallmark Channel's *Home and Family* show, who offered her tips for dressing the postbaby body earlier in this book) once brought her baby to set when her sitter flaked out at the last minute. Did the production come crashing down? No. We all helped her watch the baby while she did her job. One of my former bosses brought her little one to the office because of a childcare mix-up. Again, it worked out fine. It happens, and we all must do it at one point or another. Don't be scared of it, *own* it (especially in this day and age that pushes for more flex work for families). Share your baby with your workplace in some small way, once, if and when it's appropriate—it's the final, fake-it-to-make-it, fail-forward task for being a FAB new mom.

3 Fixes for Faking It When You're Not Feelin' It

From Debbie Matenopoulos, mom, cohost of Hallmark Channel's Home & Family, *cohost of* The Insider *on CBS, and best-selling cookbook author*

Although I've been a fan forever (hello, do you remember Debbie launching ABC's *The View* talk show way back when?), I first officially met her in 2013 when we briefly worked together on Hallmark Channel's *Home & Family*—before she became a mom. I was so nervous to introduce myself, but once I did, she was quite possibly the most relatable person I'd ever worked with at that time. Now, as a mom, I admire her ability to manage a most demanding schedule (hosting two national television shows!) while maintaining her strong family values in a most real way. I'm tickled pink to share Debbie's fixes for fakin' it through challenging, working mom days here.

1. **Drink up**. I know this may sound silly, but drinking cool water with cucumber, lemon, or orange slices can really rejuvenate you. I carry a bottle around and sip it all day long. Stay away from sugary complex carbohydrates; you'll get a quick rush, but you'll feel worse before you know it.
2. **Think of the end**. Most people's workday is 9 a.m. to 5 p.m. (or something similar to it). Resist approaching the day as though you're going to be there forever; there is a beginning, a middle, and an end. Start your day with the end in mind. Just like my husband says, "You've got to do it anyway, so you might as well do it with a smile on

your face!" If you need a quick pickup, go outside and walk around during lunch break—fresh air does wonders.

3. **Prepare for leftovers.** I often buy a whole chicken and can stretch three dinners from it; the first night will be chicken breast with sides, the second night will be chicken quesadillas (using leftover shredded chicken), the third night can be the remainder of the shredded chicken and bones made into a soup! If you're able to precut veggies and keep them in the fridge, none of these things will take you more than ten minutes. If you're too tired for that, then kick up your heels and order in, lady!

The Most Fabulous Finds of All.

Finally, we've made it! Your baby is almost ONE! (Are we FAB yet? Are we, are we?) Yes. We are. You are. But, here's the news flash, which might tick you off now that we've reached the end of this journey: you've been FAB this whole time. The fact that you were even interested and curious enough to open a book about bouncing back fast after baby proves you were already thinking about resilience and reinvention through new motherhood. You just needed an extra nudge to convince you to *really* go there and that going there is okay.

As you've probably figured out, this book is about empowering any and all choices you'll make as a new mom. The personal tips and tricks I shared were not complicated schemes; they were random things I tried out of desperate common sense, in the moment, to solve an issue or problem in the fastest way possible. That's another FAB tip: make choices fast (credit to my mom for teaching me this growing up). Taking care of a new baby doesn't feasibly allow anyone to take her sweet time with anything, much less problem-solve in a drawn out and completely logical way on a daily basis. Time is a new mother's most precious resource, and bouncing back depends on being honest about which choices will get you through your most challenging times with baby in the fastest, easiest way possible . . . and then *doing* them without doubt.

I've shared how I gave up on breastfeeding (before even starting), when I bought myself a piece of jewelry, and why walking around in underwear will make you powerful only to give you permission to make choices and try crazy schemes that will be right for *you and your family*. One of the hard truths about making choices, especially in this information age where there are sometimes *too many* options to choose from, is that we fear they may be not good enough or just plain irrational—being FAB means not being afraid to do what will allow you to feel like you so that you can be a kick-ass new mom.

Maybe you won't have issues with nursing and won't ever need to bust out bottles on your nightstand before bedtime. Maybe you are married to a man who will gift you with the most unbelievable bed making before he leaves the house every morning so you feel organized from the get-go. Maybe you won't experience any kind of identity shift once your baby is born. Or, maybe you now have a frank guide to find comfort and inspiration in when some of the things I've described blindside you a few months from now. What-ever your own journey entails, enjoy all the ups and downs it brings and stay on a focused track.

Another truth I must admit to: the activities I encourage you to do in this book are created for the purpose of having tangible, short-term goals to pass the time and make you feel like you're accomplishing something positive, consistently. Without small daily goals, a new mom's life can lose the spark of achievement that many of us got addicted to from working and just living life before becoming moms. Activity plus satisfaction always equals motivation (even if the activity is just swiping some lip gloss on in that kitchen mirror). Do something that makes you feel useful or happy and you'll feel an instant boost to do something more, make something better, or tackle that sleep training again. Keep your motivation active so you can get to baby's first birthday feeling like your life has been rockin' all year long.

My first daughter's first birthday back in 2011 was the day I felt like I'd "made it" as a mother. We'd invited about forty family members and friends to our house for a "Ladybug Picnic Barbeque" only to find out, after I'd sent the invitations, that I'd be assigned by CNN to interview Hugh Jackman that same morning (this was part of that long process I mentioned earlier about being up for that big job when my daughter was nine months old and I was secretly pregnant with my second). I planned and did most everything ahead of the big day—bought the food and supplies five days ahead, stuffed that piñata four days ahead, made my complicated Armenian stuffed grape leaves appetizers three days ahead, planted flowers in my patio two days ahead, and set up our decorations the night before interviewing Hugh.

I made the most of every single minute that week to prepare for the party and the final opportunity that almost landed me a huge job. That week was rough (too rough; I'll never do that again), but everything was a success—the party and my interview. I knew I'd made it. *I did it.* It was personal proof I'd bounced back: I sucked it up and handled what could've turned into a disastrous week of stress and a flop of a party. And the only reason I was able to handle it was because I'd conditioned myself to it by doing all those short goals and choices right after having my baby. You can do it, too. You *will* do it, too.

Are you going to maintain this program past year one and for future children? Maybe, but most likely not. I have more trouble maintaining much of what I've described here now that I'm six years into the motherhood game and have school-aged kids with activities and responsibilities that pull me in so many different directions. (Although I'm suddenly inspired to do some push-ups tonight against my bathroom sink . . .) The point of doing what I've suggested here within the first year of motherhood is to hit the ground running in an effort to set a solid, consistent standard for your new life as a mom from the very beginning. It's easier to get on a track, fall off it, and then get back rather than never getting on a track at all and feeling lost from the beginning. You get me?

As long as you continue to try, you're winning. (Trust me, I fall off and get back on more times that I can keep track of.) Resiliency is built by knowing how to make yourself happy and productive when you feel your own sense of security and power slipping out of your reach . . . and then *doing* what it's going to take to get your head and heart back in the game. Resiliency is about trying things again and again, in different ways, until you find what really works—even if it means getting on the same damn horse after being kicked off three times in a row. Resiliency is a life skill that carries use through parenting, work, marriage, breakups, triumph, failure, and beyond and becomes an example for our kids about what it means to cope with life as they grow. Be the example of perseverance you want to show your kids from the get-go—because once you start, it's hard to go back.

Having a baby sets us up for all the opportunity we'll ever need to become *better* in every way, by default. Pregnancy and the first year of motherhood present a once-in-a-lifetime opportunity for us to become more motivated and more resilient when babies pop into the picture, because we must become emotionally stronger to raise a happy, adjusted, and healthy child. The choice to pony up to the challenge or poop out with the diapers is up to us—*the choice to become a resilient woman and mother is yours*. If you remember one thing from this book, remember this: a true bounceback after baby is an incomparable reinvention forward that will build your skills to become a more confident parent for the future. My bounceback after babies made our toddler years (and now my kids' early school years) much less intimidating and absolutely more fun.

What's the most fabulous part about this journey? Your child will be with you as you commit to this FAB transformation; he will root for you in ways that will keep you going without even knowing it. Your baby will indirectly serve as your coach throughout what I've described tackling; she'll talk to you, she'll scream at you, she'll challenge and inspire you to figure it all out (my girls did). She'll also bless you with an ongoing happiness you never thought possible, even on those "failed" days and in those bad moments. With your baby as your driving force to becoming a better you, you might find soon find yourself grateful to his uncanny knack for kicking you in the butt, toughening you up, and pushing you to evolve into someone you could never become without him. And isn't that what life's about anyway? Evolving into someone better than we were before?

Just before becoming a mom, one of my former colleagues gave me a most deep heads-up that I think of almost every day, to this day. She said, "Once you have a baby, the stupid things in life stop bothering you—no matter what kind of awful day you have at work, no matter how much you get yelled at by your boss, or no matter how much you feel like you messed up, that baby loves you no matter what. It's empowering; it makes you more confident and capable." She was right. Things that used to make me nervous or question my own capabilities about career and relationships no longer bother me because I have babies (well, young kids now) who outclass and exceed anything that may happen or not happen in all other areas of my life. Babies give us assurance and an incomparable sense of self-worth that motivates us to be resilient through everything else!

It's been an absolute thrill taking you on this ride. Whatever challenges get hurled at you in your early parenting journey, you will be fine. You'll be better than fine—you'll be *fabulous*. Bounce forth without fear, have lots of fun, stay focused on the choices you choose, always fail forward, and always choose to bounce back big (even if it takes a few tries along the way). Do it for you and your family. Welcome to your new life, FAB mom.

ACKNOWLEDGMENTS

E very time I've thought about writing my thank-yous for this book, my heart would jump. Firstly, because naming names right here would mean that this book was done and final, and the reality of that scared me a bit. And secondly, the thought of accidentally forgetting to thank someone vital to this journey as this was going to print made me nervous. Writing this guide was a wild bucket-list idea that struck me when my first daughter was about four months old and then struck me again in 2013 when my youngest daughter turned one—it was a goal I couldn't seem to shake as years passed. I couldn't be more thankful, thrilled, and in total disbelief as I write my gratitude to the folks that have been with me on this crazy ride. Here goes nothing . . .

To my book agent, Fran Black of Literary Counsel—you've been the creative cheerleader that I looked so hard for, for so long! Thank you for believing in this book, thank you for our early strategy sessions over the phone, and thank you for taking a chance on me (even though it took me a year to get my act together). To my editor, Nicole Frail at Skyhorse Publishing—your always-patient responses to my paranoid, first-time author questions have meant so much to me. Thank you for making one of my longtime dreams (to be a published author) come true. For my talented illustrator, Anne Keenan Higgins—your gorgeous cover took my breath away, and still does! I am also grateful for the savvy smarts of Nicole Wool, Shae DeWaal, and the team at Jones Social. (Nicole, we finally got to work together!)

Thank you to the famous faces and experts who so graciously offered their insights and opinions for this project: Dr. Tanya Altmann, Jennifer Cohen, Sia Cooper, Allyson Downey, Samantha Ettus, Katie Hurley, Ali Landry, Debbie Matenopoulos, Catherine McCord, Cheryl Petran, Anya Sarre, Orly Shani, Katherine Stone—you have NO IDEA how moved I was by your immediate and enthusiastic support and contribution to this venture. For Doyin Richards: thank you not only for the advice you offer in this book, but for also being interested enough in this topic of mine to introduce me to Fran—without your contagious drive for making dreams reality, this book would've never happened. (Man, I owe you big-time!)

I want to give a huge thank-you to Bill Dallman, Pat Harvey, Steve Mauldin, Annette Zapata, and the entire on-air, producing and digital teams at CBS Los Angeles for giving this "FAB mom" a most spontaneous, remarkable, and unique opportunity (and most friendly and positive platform) to regularly tackle the ups and downs of parenting on Los Angeles television this past year— being your "FAB Mom on 2" has been one of my most favorite achievements to happen in my life. And, more major gratitude to the "news-moms" who had new babies this past year: Suzanne Marques, Stephanie Simmons, Stephanie Stanton, and Evelyn Taft. Thank you for sharing your most thoughtful tips and stories; you all know how to bounce back good!

Thank you to my extended family, old and new Southern California friends, and hometown fans and friends in Fresno, California—you keep me going and make me feel like I'm doing something valuable when I start doubting the point of all this FAB mom stuff. For the countless bloggers, writers, editors, and members of the digital-influencing community who have been so giving in supporting my work over the years (Hey guys, can you retweet and share?)—I consider you my friends in real life and am most grateful for being a part of this special "online parents club" we're all in together.

For my mom and dad—you've been the most tremendous parents and I am always beyond grateful that I was raised by you. For my mom—this "bouncing back fast" notion was your idea in the first place (back in 2010), and I feel so lucky to have been a recipient of your ongoing guidance to always "handle it" and frank opinions about so many things over the years. To my sister, Denise—what would I do without your straight-talking advice? You're the other original FAB mom (behind Mom, that is).

Leah and Samantha, you are the wild and wacky loves of my life, and I thank God every day that you found me when you did. Thank you for being you, for making me better, for being my girls. I can't wait to see how you bounce through life.

And finally, to my husband Andre: thank you for always being on board with my goals (even if they are inconvenient to family life sometimes). I appreciate you and love you for all the times you've let me do my thing. You're absolutely fabulous.

ABOUT THE AUTHOR

If you want to bounce back fast after having a baby, talk to Jill Simonian. Jill's signature, straight-talking style has become a go-to resource across media for motivating millions of moms to stay motivated in family life; mind, body and spirit.

Sharp and engaging on social media, television and her blog TheFABMom.com, Southern California television viewers affectionately know Jill from her lively and credible twice-weekly "FAB Mom" segments on CBS Los Angeles news, tackling hot topic parenting issues and modern family lifestyle challenges. Jill has additionally shared tips for staying "focused after babies" via NBC's *TODAY Show*, HLN's *The Daily Share*, Hallmark Channel's *Home & Family*, Mom.me, Babble.com, and Right Start baby stores. Jill is also a regular columnist for her hometown newspaper, the Fresno Bee.

Prior to becoming a mom, Jill worked as an entertainment journalist and TV host for CNN/HLN, Travel Channel, KTLA Los Angeles, and ReelzChannel. Jill lives in Los Angeles with her husband and two young daughters.

@jillsimonian
TheFABMom.com

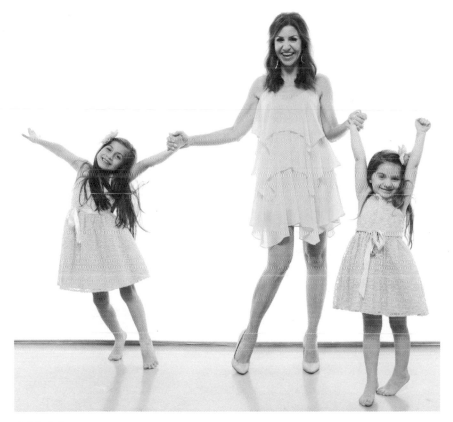